Sleep Disorders

Editor

SHAMEKA L. CODY

NURSING CLINICS
OF NORTH AMERICA

www.nursing.theclinics.com

Consulting Editor
STEPHEN D. KRAU

June 2021 • Volume 56 • Number 2

ELSEVIER

1600 John F. Kennedy Boulevard ● Suite 1800 ● Philadelphia, Pennsylvania, 19103-2899

http://www.theclinics.com

NURSING CLINICS OF NORTH AMERICA Volume 56, Number 2
June 2021 ISSN 0029-6465, ISBN-13: 978-0-323-81066-1

Editor: Kerry Holland
Developmental Editor: Axell Ivan Jade M. Purificacion

Nursing Clinics of North America (ISSN 0029-6465) is published quarterly by Elsevier Inc., 360 Park Avenue South, New York, NY 10010-1710. Months of issue are March, June, September, and December. Periodicals postage paid at New York, NY and additional mailing offices. Subscription price per year is, $163.00 (US individuals), $669.00 (US institutions), $275.00 (international individuals), $692.00 (international institutions), $231.00 (Canadian individuals), $692.00 (Canadian institutions), $100.00 (US and Canadian students), and $135.00 (international students). To receive student/resident rate, orders must be accompanied by name of affiliated institution, date of term, and the signature of program/residency coordinator on institution letterhead. Orders will be billed at individual rate until proof of status is received. Foreign air speed delivery is included in all *Clinics* subscription prices. All prices are subject to change without notice. **POSTMASTER:** Send address changes to *Nursing Clinics*, Elsevier Health Sciences Division, Subscription Customer Service, 3251 Riverport Lane, Maryland Heights, MO 63043. **Customer Service: Telephone: 1-800-654-2452** (U.S. and Canada); **1-314-447-8871 (outside U.S. and Canada). Fax: 1-314-447-8029. E-mail: journalscustomerservice-usa@elsevier.com** (for print support) and **journalsonlinesupport-usa@elsevier.com** (for online support).

Nursing Clinics of North America is covered in *EMBASE/Excerpta Medica, MEDLINE/PubMed (Index Medicus), Social Sciences Citation Index, Current Contents, ASCA, Cumulative Index to Nursing, RNdex Top 100,* and Allied Health Literature and International Nursing Index (INI).

Contributors

CONSULTING EDITOR

STEPHEN D. KRAU, PhD, RN, CNE
Associate Professor (Ret), Vanderbilt University School of Nursing, Nashville, Tennessee, USA

EDITOR

SHAMEKA L. CODY, PhD, AGNP-C
Assistant Professor, Capstone College of Nursing, The University of Alabama, Tuscaloosa, Alabama, USA

AUTHORS

KRISTI A. ACKER, DNP, PhD, FNP-BC, AOCNP, ACHPN
Clinical Assistant Professor, Capstone College of Nursing, The University of Alabama, Tuscaloosa, Alabama, USA

AMY S. BERKLEY, PhD, RN
Zimmerman Postdoctoral Fellow, University of Kansas School of Nursing, Kansas City, Kansas, USA

KATHERINE CARROLL BRITT, BSN, RN
PhD Student, The University of Texas at Austin, School of Nursing, Austin, Texas, USA

PATRICIA CARTER, PhD, RN, CNS
Professor, Assistant Dean for Graduate Programs, Capstone College of Nursing, The University of Alabama, Tuscaloosa, Alabama, USA

W. CHANCE NICHOLSON, PhD, MS, PMHNP-BC
Assistant Research Professor, Nell Hodgson Woodruff School of Nursing, Emory University, Atlanta, Georgia, USA

EILEEN R. CHASENS, PhD, RN, FAAN
Professor, School of Nursing, University of Pittsburgh, Pittsburgh, Pennsylvania, USA

SHAMEKA L. CODY, PhD, AGNP-C
Assistant Professor, Capstone College of Nursing, The University of Alabama, Tuscaloosa, Alabama, USA

SHANNON M. CONSTANTINIDES, PhD, MSN, FNP, NP-C, RN
Colorado Center of Orthopedic Excellence, Colorado Springs, Colorado, USA

NORMA CUELLAR, PhD, RN, FAAN
Professor, The University of Alabama, Tuscaloosa, Alabama, USA

MONICA M. DINARDO, PhD, ANP-BC, CDCES
Health Science Specialist, Center for Heath Equity Research and Promotion, VA
Pittsburgh Healthcare System, Pittsburgh, Pennsylvania, USA

SANDRA ESTES, EdD, MSN
Clinical Assistant Professor, Capstone College of Nursing, The University of Alabama,
Project Manager, Tuscaloosa Veterans Affairs Medical Center, Tuscaloosa Research and
Education Advancement Corporation, Tuscaloosa, Alabama, USA

CASSANDRA M. GODZIK, PhD, APRN
Postdoctoral Research Fellow, Department of Psychiatry, Dartmouth College and
Dartmouth-Hitchcock Medical Center, Lebanon, New Hampshire, USA

KAREN HEATON, PhD, COHN-S, FNP-BC, FAAN, FAAOHN
Associate Professor and Coordinator of PhD Program, Director, Department of Acute,
Chronic and Continuing Care, The University of Alabama at Birmingham School of
Nursing, Birmingham, Alabama, USA

SAMANTHA V. HILL, MD, MPH
Assistant Professor, Department of Pediatrics, Division of Adolescent Medicine, The
University of Alabama at Birmingham, Birmingham, Alabama, USA

CHRISTOPHER C. IMES, PhD, RN
Assistant Professor, School of Nursing, University of Pittsburgh, Pittsburgh,
Pennsylvania, USA

BOMIN JEON, MSN, RN, PhD Candidate
Predoctoral Student, School of Nursing, University of Pittsburgh, Pittsburgh,
Pennsylvania, USA

JACOB K. KARIUKI, PhD, AGNP-BC
Assistant Professor, School of Nursing, University of Pittsburgh, Pittsburgh,
Pennsylvania, USA

ABIGAIL KAZEMBE, PhD, RN
Associate Professor, Neonatal and Reproductive Health Services, Kamuzu College of
Nursing, The University of Malawi, Lilongwe, Malawi

MANGALA KRISHNAMURTHY, MLIS, AHIP
Reference Librarian/Associate Professor, Rodgers Science and Engineering Library, The
University of Alabama Libraries, Tuscaloosa, Alabama, USA

FAITH S. LUYSTER, PhD
Assistant Professor, School of Nursing, University of Pittsburgh, Pittsburgh,
Pennsylvania, USA

GIBRAN MANCUS, PhD, RN
Assistant Professor, Capstone College of Nursing, The University of Alabama,
Tuscaloosa, Alabama, USA

LAURIE A. MARTINEZ, PhD, MBA, MSN, RN
Florida Atlantic University, Christine E. Lynn College of Nursing, Boca Raton, Florida, USA

JONNA L. MORRIS, PhD, RN
Assistant Professor, School of Nursing, University of Pittsburgh, Pittsburgh,
Pennsylvania, USA

JANET MORRISON, PhD, RN
Project Director, The University of Texas at Austin, School of Nursing, Austin, Texas, USA

MARÍA DE LOS ÁNGELES ORDÓÑEZ, DNP, APRN, GNP-BC, PMHNP-BC, CDP, FAANP, FAAN
Director, Associate Professor, Member, FAU Memory Disorder Clinic Coordinator, Associate Professor, Louis and Anne Green Memory and Wellness Center of the Christine E. Lynn College of Nursing (CELCON), Florida Atlantic University (FAU), Alzheimer's Disease Initiative, Florida Department of Elder Affairs, Federal Advisory Council on Alzheimer's Research, Care, and Services, US Department of Health and Human Services, Boca Raton, Florida, USA

PATRICIA DE LOS ÁNGELES ORDÓÑEZ, MS, CDP
Psychology Trainee (Clinical Psychology), FAU Assistant Memory Disorder Clinic Coordinator, Nova Southeastern University (NSU), College of Psychology, Care, Supportive Services, and Outreach Coordinator, Louis and Anne Green Memory, Wellness Center of the Christine E. Lynn College of Nursing (CELCON), Florida Atlantic University (FAU), Alzheimer's Disease Initiative, Florida Department of Elder Affairs, Associate Professor of the Christine E. Lynn College of Nursing at Florida Atlantic University, Assistant Professor of Clinical Biomedical Science (Secondary) of the Charles E. Schmidt College of Medicine at Florida Atlantic University, Davie, Florida, USA

PAMELA PAYNE-FOSTER, MD, MPH
Professor, College of Community Health Sciences, The University of Alabama, Tuscaloosa, Alabama, USA

KATE PFEIFFER, MSN, PMHNP-BC, PMHCNS-BC
Instructor, Nell Hodgson Woodruff School of Nursing, Emory University, Atlanta, Georgia, USA

SHAMEKA PHILLIPS, MSN, FNP-C
PhD Nursing Student, UAB Nutrition and Obesity Research Center (NORC), Pre-Doctoral Fellow, The University of Alabama at Birmingham School of Nursing, Birmingham, Alabama, USA

KATHY RICHARDS, PhD, RN, FAAN
Senior Research Scientist and Research Professor, The University of Texas at Austin, School of Nursing, Austin, Texas, USA

JENNIFER M. ROURKE, MS, RN, AGCNS-BC, CCRN
Critical Care Clinical Nurse Specialist, VA Portland Health Care System, Portland, Oregon, USA

JOHNNY R. TICE, DNP, MA, CRNP, FNP-C, PMHNP-BC
Clinical Assistant Professor, Capstone College of Nursing, The University of Alabama, Tuscaloosa, Alabama, USA

YANYAN WANG, PhD
Research Associate, The University of Texas at Austin, School of Nursing, Austin, Texas, USA

TERESA M. WARD, RN, PhD, FAAN
Professor, Department of Child, Family, and Population Health Nursing, University of Washington School of Nursing, Seattle, Washington, USA

KRIS B. WEYMANN, PhD, RN
Assistant Professor of Clinical Nursing, Nurse Scientist, VA Portland Health Care System, Oregon Health & Science University, School of Nursing, Portland, Oregon, USA

YOLANDA SMITH WHEELER, PhD, CRNP, CPNP-AC, MSCN
Assistant Professor, Department of Family, Community and Health Systems, The University of Alabama at Birmingham School of Nursing, UAB Center for Pediatric Onset Demyelinating Disease, Birmingham, Alabama, USA

KYEONGRA YANG, PhD, MPH, RN
Associate Professor, School of Nursing, Rutgers, The State University of New Jersey, Newark, New Jersey, USA

SHUMENGHUI ZHAI, MPH
PhD Student, University of Washington School of Nursing, Seattle, Washington, USA

Contents

Sleep and Immune Function

> Sleep is a critical issue for quality of life, cognition, and safety among patients with MS. Sleep disturbances from poor sleep hygiene, and multiple sclerosis symptomology, sleep disorders are prevalent; yet evaluation of sleep and screening of sleep disorders are inconsistent. This article presents commonly observed sleep disturbances and disorders, appropriate screening and diagnostic considerations, and management options. Nurses providing care for patients with MS must recognize sleep as an important component in care planning. A comprehensive sleep history and appropriate screening instruments should be incorporated into initial and ongoing assessments, with referral to sleep medicine providers as indicated.

> Sleep-wake disturbances are common in patients with cancer. Despite the high prevalence of altered sleep patterns in oncology settings, there remains a gap in consistent assessment of sleep, leading to an underrecognized and undertreated condition. Provider failure in addressing sleep-wake disturbances can result in chronic issues with insomnia and has a negative impact on quality of life and cancer survivorship. Often sleep-wake disturbances present in symptom "clusters" including, anxiety, depression, and fatigue, which adds to the complexity of managing sleep disorders in oncology. Aggressive management strategies for managing underlying symptom burden from disease or medications effects is a priority.

> Following diagnosis of human immunodeficiency virus (HIV), getting adequate sleep may be the farthest thing from the mind of patients or providers. Even further from mind are the potential benefits on both sleep and HIV from nature-based therapy. In developing and developed countries, access to high-quality natural spaces has the potential to support physical and mental health. This article provides a review of sleep disorders, conventional and nature-based therapies, and the potential of nature-based

therapy to support the health of people living with HIV through increased restorative sleep and immune function.

Sleep and Inflammation

Metabolic syndrome (MetS) refers to the clustering of risk factors for cardiovascular disease and diabetes, including central adiposity, hypertension, dyslipidemia, and hyperglycemia. During the past 20 years, there have been parallel and epidemic increases in MetS and impaired sleep. This article describes evidence on the association between MetS and short sleep duration, circadian misalignment, insomnia, and sleep apnea. Potential mechanisms where impaired sleep desynchronizes and worsens metabolic control and interventions to improve sleep and potentially improve MetS are presented.

Sleep and Mental Health

 Video content accompanies this article at http://www.nursing.theclinics.com.

Veterans are those who have served our country in one of the branches of armed forces or military reserves. The Veterans Health Administration is the largest integrated health system in the nation, providing health care services and latest research for veterans. Non–Veteran Health Administration primary care clinicians, who also take care of veterans, deserve to have an understanding of the unique challenges and conditions these individuals face and the resources that are available to improve sleep health and well-being of all veterans. This article guides these clinicians to manage sleep disorders, mental health disorders, and substance use among veterans.

Sleep disruptions are frequently reported by persons with mood, anxiety, and post-traumatic stress disorders, and co-occur with psychiatric disorders. There is evidence that sleep disorders can predict the likelihood of developing a future psychiatric disorder and exacerbate existing symptoms. Understanding the inter-relationships between sleep and psychiatric disorders is important. The primary goals of this article are to describe the interactions between psychiatric and sleep disorders in the context of sleep disturbances, underscore the bidirectional effects of mental health treatments on sleep disorder outcomes, and provide general recommendations to optimize treatment in the context of sleep disturbances.

Sleep and Neurological Disorders

Over a typical lifespan, the amount of time people spend each day sleeping decreases. Sleep patterns also change as people age. Sleep disorders are common among persons of all ages, and older adults are particularly vulnerable. Development of age-related neurodegenerative diseases, such as Alzheimer's disease and related dementias, is associated with pronounced sleep disruption. This article provides evidence-based guidelines for diagnosis and clinical management of sleep disorders that occur during the course of treatment of Alzheimer's disease and related dementias. The article presents novel interventions and future directions for clinical practice and sleep research, and addresses diversity and inclusivity.

Restless legs syndrome (RLS), one of the more prevalent sleep disturbances among older adults, impacts quality of life. Patients with dementia are at high risk for developing RLS and may be unable to describe their symptoms. Often underdiagnosed, RLS can contribute to discomfort, pain, nighttime agitation, disturbed sleep, and falls. Clinical assessment is crucial and should include a thorough evaluation with input from the patient and family, deprescribing medication if possible, and consideration of common sleep-disturbing factors. Evidence-based treatment in this population is limited; overall focus should center on relieving discomfort while identifying and treating bothersome sleep symptoms.

Sleep disturbances are common after traumatic brain injury of all levels of severity, interfere with acute and long-term recovery, and can persist for years after injury. There is increasing evidence of the importance of sleep in improving brain function and recovery. Noticing and addressing sleep disturbances are important aspects of nursing care, especially for the prevention or early recognition of delirium. Nonpharmacologic interventions can improve sleep. Teaching about the importance of sleep after traumatic brain injury, promoting sleep hygiene, and multidisciplinary approaches to addressing sleep problems and improving sleep are important for recovery from traumatic brain injury.

Sleep and Physiological Function

Older adults who do not sleep well frequently have difficulty sustaining attention, display slower physical response times, and have memory issues that may contribute to depression or early dementia. The life changes that accompany aging, such as retirement, bereavement, or the onset of chronic illness or disability, can precipitate sleep problems. Insomnia and obstructive sleep apnea are the most common sleep disorders in older adults and can have far-reaching consequences on health and well-being. Nurses should include thorough sleep assessments in any patient interview.

The breadth of childhood sleep problems is broad and can be associated with biologic, psychiatric, behavioral, social, and environmental processes. Unrecognized childhood sleep problems may threaten daytime behaviors and negatively impact school and psychosocial functioning. Left unattended, overall child biopsychosocial development may be impaired. Thus, identifying and addressing sleep problems has potential to optimize childhood health, development, and overall well-being. Nurses need to be cognizant of detrimental impacts of child sleep deprivation and advocate for appropriate sleep assessments while offering sleep education to parents and children.

Sleep and Chronic Pain

Sleep deficiency in children is a public health concern, and it is highly comorbid in pediatric chronic pain conditions. Children may be particularly vulnerable to the deleterious effects of sleep deficiency, because comorbid sleep deficiency in chronic pain may further exacerbate already existent symptoms of pain, anxiety, depressions, daytime function, and increase health care use. Sleep deficiency is modifiable and integrating human-centered approaches into the development of sleep interventions is a pragmatic approach to partner with parents and children to provide them with the knowledge, motivation, and skills for setting and achieving goals, adapting to setbacks, and problem solving.

NURSING CLINICS OF NORTH AMERICA

SERIES OF RELATED INTEREST

Critical Care Nursing Clinics of North America
https://www.ccnursing.theclinics.com/
Advances in Family Practice Nursing
http://www.advancesinfamilypracticenursing.com/

THE CLINICS ARE AVAILABLE ONLINE!
Access your subscription at:
www.theclinics.com

Preface

Managing Sleep Disorders with Chronic Illnesses Across the Lifespan

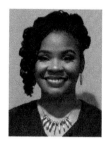

Shameka L. Cody, PhD, AGNP-C
Editor

Poor sleep is no longer considered just a symptom of chronic illness; poor sleep is now viewed as a consequence of chronic illness. The documented adverse effects of not getting enough sleep or having a poor quality of sleep include fatigue, irritability, poor concentration, poor work and school performance, driving and occupational-related injuries, depression, and poor quality of life. Patient reports of sleeping problems may be a precursor to an underlying medical condition or exacerbated by treatment of a current health condition. As the general population continues to age with chronic illnesses that were once short lived, routine sleep assessments are critical for early diagnosis and treatment of sleep disorders. Manifestations of sleep disorders among patients with chronic illnesses can differ across the lifespan, and such differences necessitate clinical strategies to prevent a delay in diagnosis and treatment.

The Centers for Disease Control and Prevention has declared sleep disorders a public health issue given its association with chronic health conditions and increased morbidity and mortality. Nurses provide care for patients with sleep disorders across the lifespan in various health care settings. This special issue of *Nursing Clinics of North America* on sleep disorders provides a cross-section of works as they apply to patients with chronic illnesses across the lifespan. The review articles provide evidence-based guidelines for assessing sleep health during infancy through older adulthood in patients with chronic immunologic, psychological, and physiologic conditions (**Fig. 1**). Many of the review articles in this issue present clinical case studies that highlight challenges related to diagnosing and treating sleep disorders that coexist with chronic illnesses. It is hoped this issue will guide clinicians to inquire more about sleeping problems and use a comprehensive approach to treating sleep disorders. The lack of attention to sleep disorders is detrimental to patient health outcomes,

https://doi.org/10.1016/j.cnur.2021.03.003
0029-6465/21/© 2021 Published by Elsevier Inc.
nursing.theclinics.com

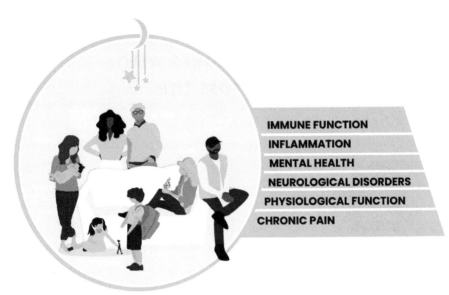

Fig. 1. Sleep disorders with chronic illnesses across the lifespan. (Created by Kellie Hensley.)

especially during the COVID-19 pandemic, when consequences of sleep disorders may be more severe and impede recovery.

Special thanks to Dr Patricia Carter (Professor and Assistant Dean of Graduate Programs, Capstone College of Nursing, The University of Alabama), Dr Suzanne Prevost (Dean and Professor at Capstone College of Nursing, The University of Alabama), Kellie Hensley (graphic designer), and contributing authors.

Shameka L. Cody, PhD, AGNP-C
Capstone College of Nursing
The University of Alabama
Box 870358
Tuscaloosa, AL 35487, USA

E-mail address:
slcody@ua.edu

Sleep and Immune Function

Distinguishing the Diagnosis and Management of Sleep Disturbance and Sleep Disorders in Multiple Sclerosis

Yolanda Smith Wheeler, PhD, CRNP, CPNP-AC, MSCN[a],*,
Karen Heaton, PhD, COHN-S, FNP-BC, FAAOHN[b]

KEYWORDS

- Multiple sclerosis • Sleep disturbance • Sleep disorders

KEY POINTS

- The pathophysiology of multiple sclerosis, the nature of the disease process, and the management of acute and ongoing symptoms complicate the diagnosis and management of sleep disturbance in patients with multiple sclerosis.
- The management of multiple sclerosis symptoms like pain, fatigue, and bladder and bowel dysfunction by a multidisciplinary team must be addressed along with good sleep hygiene to improve sleep quality in patients with multiple sclerosis.
- If a sleep disorder is suspected, initial and periodic screening are necessary to ensure appropriate evaluation, management, and treatment of the disorder.

INTRODUCTION

Multiple sclerosis (MS) is an autoimmune disorder of the central nervous system (CNS) that affects the brain, spinal cord, optic nerves, and the CNS pathway. The average disease onset is between 20 and 40 years, with a mean age of approximately 30 years.[1] However, it is known that MS can affect a person of any age. Of individuals with MS, 3% to 5% are estimated to be less than 18 years of age and an estimated 4% to 9% of individuals are rarely diagnosed with late onset MS after the age of 50.[2–4] Women are affected 2 to 3 times more than men and the highest prevalence

[a] Department of Family, Community and Health Systems, University of Alabama at Birmingham (UAB) School of Nursing, UAB Center for Pediatric Onset Demyelinating Disease, 1720 2nd Avenue South, NB 450, Birmingham, AL 35294-1210, USA; [b] Department of Acute, Chronic & Continuing Care, UAB School of Nursing, 1720 2nd Avenue South, NB 450, Birmingham, AL 35294-1210, USA
* Corresponding author.
E-mail address: yowheeler@uab.edu
Twitter: @Yolanda67445802 (Y.S.W.)

Nurs Clin N Am 56 (2021) 157–174
https://doi.org/10.1016/j.cnur.2021.02.001
0029-6465/21/Published by Elsevier Inc.
nursing.theclinics.com

is in North America.[1] The most recent MS prevalence study estimated the total number of people affected in the United States to be 1 million.[5]

It is believed that individuals who are diagnosed with MS have a genetic predisposition followed by an environmental trigger that causes the degradation of myelin sheath and a breakdown of the blood–brain barrier, causing the formation of lesions in brain matter, the spinal cord, and the optic nerves. The immune response leads to inflammation, demyelination, axonal loss, and eventually physical and cognitive disability over time.[6] Lesions or plaques on the brain, spinal cord and optic nerves are identified by MRI and cause an interruption of communication between the neural pathways, which manifests as symptoms. MS is a diagnosis of exclusion; there is no 1 test that can be given to make a diagnosis of MS. Laboratory testing and comparison of serial examination and MRI imaging rule out differential diagnoses. An MS diagnosis is made by sorting out the clinical symptoms and evidence that suggests that there is no other condition likely using the McDonald criteria, a diagnostic instrument used in diagnosing MS. An individual meets the McDonald criteria for MS when there is a dissemination in the accumulation of lesions seen on MRI in the spinal cord, brain, and/or optic nerves and a documented history of clinical relapse that occurs over time.[7] Although there is no cure for MS, there are currently 21 brand-name and generic medications used to modify the course of the disease and to slow the progression to permanent and irreversible disability.[8]

PATHOPHYSIOLOGY OF MULTIPLE SCLEROSIS–RELATED TO SLEEP ISSUES

The most common phenotype of MS is relapsing remitting, in which the person experiences intermittent symptoms followed by periods of little or no disease activity. There is high variability in the symptoms a person experiences, the course of the disease, and the rate of relapse for each individual based on the location and extent of the CNS damage.[9] Sleep issues in the MS population have gained recognition in the literature over the last decade; however, clinicians and health care providers rarely address this topic for individuals with the diagnosis. The literature suggests that the prevalence of individuals diagnosed with MS with some form of sleep difficulty ranges from 25% to 54%.[10,11]

There are several known factors regarding the pathophysiology of MS as it relates to sleep dysfunction. MS lesions that accumulate and neural damage to key structures like the hypothalamus and brain stem can lead to sleep disorders like hypersomnia, narcolepsy, and sleep apnea. The hypothalamus is the area of the brain responsible for many physiologic processes, one of which is the sleep–rest cycle. The brain stem regulates breathing and involuntary nerve function during sleep.[12] If lesions or damage from MS occur in these 2 areas of the brain, then the person may have difficulty maintaining a sleep–wake cycle, have disruptions in breathing during sleep, or suffer from a sleep disorder. Lesions in the dorsal pontine tegmentum and medulla can lead to REM sleep behavior disorders or sleep-related breathing disorders. In addition, periodic limb movement disorder is due to infratentorial lesions within the cerebellum, brain stem, and spinal cord, and restless leg syndrome is indicated in upper spinal cord lesions.[12]

In addition, there is a disruption of key neurotransmitters that may also cause narcolepsy, fatigue, or the improper regulation of the sleep–wake cycle. Hypocretin, a molecule produced by the hypothalamus that helps to regulate arousal, can cause narcolepsy or hypersomnia if the levels are low in an analysis of the cerebrospinal fluid.[13,14] In addition, a disruption in the neural pathways of dopamine and norepinephrine, which play an important part in cognition, movement, and motivation, can explain a person experiencing fatigue, which may be misinterpreted as sleep dysfunction.[15] Low levels of melatonin, another neurohormone involved in the sleep–wake cycle, has also been associated with poor sleep and MS relapse in recent data.[16,17]

DISTINGUISHING BETWEEN SLEEP DISTURBANCE AND SLEEP DISORDER

For the purposes of this article, sleep disturbance will be distinguished from sleep disorder. Sleep disturbance will be defined as an interruption in a person's normal sleep pattern. This interruption may be secondary to common MS symptoms. Sleep disturbance may also be the result of medications side effects or psychological problems like anxiety and depression secondary to the disease.[17] Sleep disturbance, commonly seen in MS, causes poor sleep quality, interruption in the normal sleep cycle, and leads to poor quality of life. Sleep disturbance also has the potential to have negative long-term health care outcomes and increase risk of developing comorbid conditions like diabetes, cardiac disease, and obesity.[18,19]

In contrast, a sleep disorder will be defined as an altered sleep pattern owing to the direct impact of the pathophysiology of the disease. Some of the most common sleep disorders seen in MS include hypersomnia, restless legs/body syndrome, obstructive sleep apnea, and insomnia.[20] Sleep issues, whether classified by definition of a disturbance or disorder, are seen more often in the MS population than in the general population, with estimates ranging from 25% to 54%.[10,11,21]

REVIEW OF MULTIPLE SCLEROSIS–RELATED SYMPTOMS CAUSING SLEEP DISTURBANCE

A person with MS may experience a variety of symptoms with a relapse. These symptoms may be temporary, lasting less than 6 months after an acute relapse occurs, or permanent and lasting well after the acute illness has occurred, with irreversible effects. Symptoms of MS can include impaired mobility, gait disturbance, spasticity, tremor and speech impairment, altered sensation, cognition, emotional changes, bladder and bowel dysfunction, difficulty swallowing, and vision changes, as well as fatigue. All of the symptoms that individuals with MS experience can interfere with daily functioning and quality of life.[22] Most, if not all, of the symptoms have secondary effects that interfere with and disrupt sleep.[23] The cause of poor sleep in individuals with MS is typically multifactorial with common causes including nocturia, pain, anxiety, depression, migraine, and spasms. Furthermore, if the symptoms are untreated, they may exacerbate other symptoms.[24] For example, neurogenic bladder in MS owing to lesions located in the thoracic spine can result in sleep deprivation. The individual will experience nocturia because of bladder urgency and frequency. In addition, if a person who has a neurogenic bladder has a significant level of physical disability, then the individual can also suffer from exhaustion and daytime sleepiness because of the frequency of the times a patient is required to get out bed.

Another example is neuropathic pain or musculoskeletal pain in MS. Musculoskeletal pain is a frequent finding in individuals diagnosed with MS who have spinal cord lesions. Pain in MS is cited as the main cause of initial insomnia in recent studies and is reported in one-third to one-half of people diagnosed with MS.[25] The pain that is experienced may be acute and chronic and is often associated with tonic muscle spasms, burning and aching sensations, and spasticity. Other forms of pain cited in the literature are back pain, trigeminal neuralgia, Lhermitte's sign, and headaches.[12,25] Pain related to MS originates from the sensory pathways in either the brain stem and spine, the pyramidal tracts, or the gray matter within the brain. A list of specific MS symptoms and their secondary effects are provided in **Table 1**.

Table 1	
Secondary effects of MS symptoms	
MS Symptom	**Secondary Effect**
Impaired mobility	Muscle weakness, fatigue, spasticity, loss of balance, sensory deficit, fall risk
Spasticity	Muscle spasms, pain, muscle cramps, restless limbs
Fatigue	Daytime drowsiness, decreased physical activity, impaired cognition
Pain (neuropathic/musculoskeletal)	Insomnia, fatigue, muscle weakness
Depression	Fatigue, sleepiness, insomnia, cognitive dysfunction
Anxiety	Insomnia, restlessness, fatigue
Bladder dysfunction	Nocturia, bladder incontinence
Bowel disturbance	Bowel incontinence, abdominal pain
Heat/cold intolerance	Fatigue, decreased activity, sleep disruption, temperature disruption
Sexual dysfunction	Insomnia, depression, anxiety

Medications used to treat acute symptoms and long-term management of MS can also be the cause of sleep disturbances. Corticosteroids, which are used during acute MS relapse to decrease inflammation, can cause temporary insomnia and sleeplessness because it is often given in high dosages of 500 to 1000 mg/d for 3 to 5 days.[24] In addition, interferons, considered a first-line treatment for MS, elicit flulike symptoms in most people who use them for long-term therapy.[24] Most clinicians and health professors caring for individuals on these therapies recommend giving the injections during the night to prevent the side effects of the medications. There is evidence that interferons may cause the dysregulation of melatonin, which may interrupt the sleep–wake cycle.[24] Other medications used to manage the symptoms of MS like antidepressants and antispasmodics can also cause secondary sleep disturbances. A list of prescribed medications used in the management of MS-related symptoms and their associated sleep effects is presented in **Box 1**.

The consequences of poor sleep include fatigue, excessive daytime sleepiness, altered memory and mood, pain, impaired concentration, and learning deficits, as well as anxiety and depression.[19,26] Poor sleep in a person with MS can negatively influence quality of life, causing a low functional health status and ultimately increasing the risk of mortality related to MS. Poor sleep can also increase risks of developing other coexisting conditions such as diabetes, obesity, and heart disease.[19]

REVIEW OF THE RELATIONSHIP BETWEEN SLEEP AND FATIGUE

Fatigue is defined as a lack of energy or a feeling of exhaustion that cannot be fully explained by any other symptom, such as depression or muscle weakness.[27] Fatigue is the most common and disabling symptom of MS in adults and children. Adults with MS who experience chronic fatigue or extreme fatigue often retire early or reduce their hours at their job owing to their inability to keep up with their duties while experiencing these symptoms.[28] MS-related fatigue has been reported in more than 80% of adult patients and 30% of children with MS complain of fatigue that significantly limits daily activities.[29–31]

The cause of MS fatigue is not well-established. Primary fatigue can be related to the pathophysiology of MS that results in demyelination and axonal loss secondary

Box 1		
Medications Prescribed in MS that Affect Sleep		
Medication	**Indication for Use**	**Effect on Sleep**
Ampyra	Increase walking speed	Insomnia
Corticosteroids	Acute relapse	Insomnia
Amantadine	Chronic fatigue	Insomnia
Modafinil		
Baclofen	Spasticity	Sedation, daytime sleepiness
Tizanidine	Neuropathic pain	
Gabapentin		
Diazepam		
Clonazepam		
Beta interferon	Reduce relapse rate and slow progression of MS	Insomnia, daytime sleepiness
Clonazepam	Tremor	Sleepiness
Gabapentin		
Primidone		
Propranolol		
Levetiracetam		
Topiramate		
Oxybutynin	Neurogenic bladder	Sedation, drowsiness

to high lesion load, brain atrophy, or abnormal cervical functioning. In contrast, secondary fatigue is related to frequently encountered symptoms in MS, like depression, cognitive deficits, disability, sleepiness, and pain.[32] The side effects of disease-modifying therapies and symptomatic treatments for conditions like muscle spasms and spasticity can also attribute to a person's fatigability.[24]

It is often difficult to distinguish between MS fatigue and sleepiness that is due to a sleep disturbance.[33] Sleep disorders that are undiagnosed and untreated in the MS population can also contribute to MS fatigue. Most of the studies published on sleep disturbance as a contributor to fatigue were inconclusive in distinguishing whether one phenomenon precedes the another, but found that the 2 were intertwined.[34] Most of the literature on sleep disorders and disturbance in MS supports that notion that fatigue improves as issues with sleep are properly addressed and managed.

IDENTIFYING SLEEP DISTURBANCE CAUSED BY MULTIPLE SCLEROSIS–RELATED SYMPTOMS

Managing sleep disturbance owing to MS-related symptoms is challenging. Proper identification of the underlying cause of sleep disturbance should be made. For example, if disturbed sleep occurs owing to mitigating factors like trips to the bathroom secondary to bladder or bowel dysfunction, then these issues need to be addressed. If the individual has not been prescribed medication for these issues, then a referral to a urologist or gastroenterologist is needed to determine the reason for the dysfunction (eg, incomplete emptying, urgency, etc). Once the mechanism of dysfunction is determined, then the appropriate medication or intervention can be prescribed or implemented.

Medications and substances used in the management of MS symptoms that can affect sleep include anticholinergics, stimulants, steroids, pain, spasticity, blood pressure, and headaches, as well as depression and anxiety.[33] Most patients experience more than 1 symptom simultaneously and may have a variety of pharmacologic reg-imens in place to decrease the number of symptoms experienced. The interaction of these regimens may influence sleep quality.[33]

Furthermore, conditions like insomnia worsens symptom of depression and vice versa.[17,35] MS-related neuropathic or musculoskeletal pain have also been noted more frequently in poor sleepers and cited as the main causes of initial insomnia in pa-tients with MS.[25] Other conditions like loss of activity, temperature dysregulation, sex-ual dysfunction, and spasticity should be addressed as well. These conditions may also deter quality sleep. Alcohol, tobacco, and caffeine can also impede quality sleep as well. In addition, sleep disturbance may be sign of other coexisting conditions that have occurred along with MS.

TREATING AND MANAGING SLEEP DISTURBANCE RELATED TO SYMPTOMS OF MULTIPLE SCLEROSIS

In addition to addressing MS symptoms that interfere with sleep accordingly, individ-uals with MS can improve the quality of their sleep by establishing good sleep hygiene by taking the following steps:

- Avoiding and minimize daytime naps.
- Avoid stimulant use or high carbohydrate foods close to bedtime.
- Promote natural light.
- Establish a bedtime routine.
- Adjust the temperature of the room.
- Avoid noise.
- Talk with sleep partner about room modifications.
- Use the bedroom for sleeping only.
- Establish a regular exercise routine.
- Avoid screen time close to bedtime.[36]

Also, the administration time of immunotherapies (ie, interferon) used to treat the progression of MS may be modified to improve sleep quality in individuals being treated with these regimens. Although clinicians and health care providers typically instruct patients with MS to administer these medications at night so that they can sleep through the symptoms like fever and chills, it is thought that switching the time of administration improved the quality of sleep.[37,38]

Oral and intravenous corticosteroids used to treat MS relapses can also cause tem-porary insomnia and daytime sleepiness, but resolve after the completion of the treat-ment.[39] Clinicians should advise the administration of steroid treatments in the morning to prevent sleep disturbance. The adjustment of stimulant medications pre-scribed to treat fatigue (ie, modafinil, amantadine, and methylphenidate) can be adjusted in dosage and administration time to mitigate sleep disruption.[39] The person with MS should consider having a discussion with their clinical and/or pharmacists regarding medication interactions and unwanted side effects among their prescribed, over-the-counter and complementary and alternative medications that may be the cause of fatigue or nighttime sleeplessness. Individuals with MS should also have a primary care clinician or internist to adequately assess and treat common comorbid conditions they may be experiencing along with MS.

If the individual with MS is experiencing excessive daytime drowsiness, snoring, or headaches or hoarseness in the morning, an evaluation from a health care profes-sional is warranted because these signs may indicate a sleep disorder. Additional signs that may include the individual not feeling restored or refreshed after adequate sleep or if the person is experiencing trouble falling or staying asleep after modifications to symptom management have been made.

DIAGNOSIS AND MANAGEMENT OF MULTIPLE SCLEROSIS–RELATED SLEEP DISORDERS

As stated elsewhere in this article, MS-related sleep disorders often emerge as lesions develop in specific areas of the brain and spinal cord. **Fig. 1** illustrates sleep disorders and the areas of CNS affected for each one. For the purposes of this article, 4 of the most common sleep disorders associated with MS will be discussed: Sleep-disordered breathing, restless leg syndrome, narcolepsy, and insomnia.

Sleep-Disordered Breathing

Both obstructive and central sleep apnea are associated with MS.[40] However, the prevalence, etiologies, and clinical presentations may differ when comparing persons with MS and sleep-disordered breathing with those in the general population without MS, but who have sleep-disordered breathing. For this reason, an understanding of the differences in presentation and appropriate screening and diagnostic tools are essential for the clinician working with patients with MS.

Obstructive Sleep Apnea

Obstructive sleep apnea is characterized by collapse of the upper airway, which decreases airflow and is associated with oxygen desaturation that repeats throughout the sleep period.[41] Associated symptoms and signs include excessive daytime

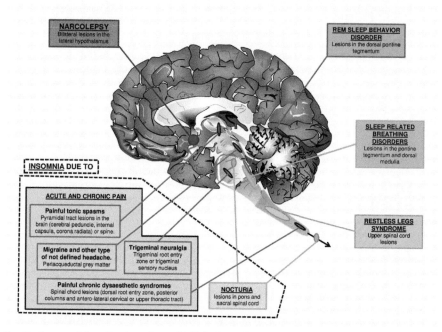

Fig. 1. Summarizing the location of MS lesions that are associated with sleep disorders. (*From* Foschi M, Rizzo G, Liguori R, et al. Sleep-related disorders and their relationship with MRI findings in multiple sclerosis. Sleep Med. 2019 Apr;56:90-97. doi: 10.1016/j.sleep.2019.01.010. Epub 2019 Jan 21.; with permission.)

sleepiness, snoring, witnessed apneas by bed partners, increased propensity for sleep in certain contexts (after meals, during meetings, etc), and, possibly, falling asleep at the wheel while driving.[42] Among the most commonly used screening instruments are STOP-BANG and the Berlin Sleep Apnea Questionnaire.[43]

The most commonly used metric for diagnosis of obstructive sleep apnea is the apnea/hypopnea index, or the number of respiratory disturbances experienced per hour. This measure is obtained via polysomnogram. The severity of obstructive sleep apnea is defined at thresholds of the apnea/hypopnea index of 5 or greater, 15, or 30, representing mild, moderate, and severe obstructive sleep apnea, respectively. In the general population, if the threshold of the apnea/hypopnea index of 5 or more is applied, obstructive sleep apnea prevalence ranges from 9% to 38%. In this group, the prevalence is typically higher in men, increases with aging, and is associated with increased body mass index and neck circumference.[44] In contrast, in the MS population, obstructive sleep apnea is prevalent, but the extent of the disorder in the population is difficult to determine because of methodologic variations in the studies conducted to date. Estimates of obstructive sleep apnea reported in patients with MS range between 36% and 56%.[45] Although MS is more prevalent in women, compared with men, obstructive sleep apnea among patients with MS is more prevalent among male patients. Similar to the general population, increased body mass index is associated with obstructive sleep apnea in patients with MS; however, there are several studies that identify obstructive sleep apnea among patients with MS with a body mass index in the mid to low 20s range.[19,45,46]

In additional to a complete history, including a comprehensive medication and substance use history, the clinician should include questions regarding sleep in the history taking. Patients should be asked questions related to snoring, daytime sleepiness, and falling asleep at inopportune times and at the wheel. A body mass index and neck circumference should be obtained as part of the physical examination. Any patient who responds positively to the history, with or without obesity and a neck circumferences of 16 cm or greater in women and 17 cm or greater in men, should be screened for obstructive sleep apnea using an instrument such as STOP-Bang.[47] Along with STOP-Bang, the Epworth Sleepiness Scale is commonly used to identify excessive daytime sleepiness, and the Fatigue Severity Scale is used to identify and differentiate fatigue from sleepiness.[43,48]

Patients who score 3 or higher on the STOP-Bang instrument are at an increased risk for obstructive sleep apnea and should be referred for overnight polysomnography.[49] The diagnosis of obstructive sleep apnea is made in the presence of apneas and/or hypopneas with decreased airflow and oxygen desaturation while the patient continues to make efforts to breathe. This contrasts with central sleep apnea, during which decreased airflow and desaturation occur, because the patient does not make efforts to breathe.[50]

Central Sleep Apnea

As mentioned elsewhere in this article, central sleep apnea occurs when both airflow and respiratory effort cease or airflow decreases as respiratory effort ceases. This pattern may also repeat throughout the sleep period and may also occur along with obstructive sleep apnea (mixed apnea) The prevalence of this condition in patients with MS is unknown, but it is seen more commonly in patients with MS with brain stem and spinal cord lesions.[40] It may also result from the use of certain medications and substances, such as opioids, medications used for the treatment of spasticity, and other sedating medications or substances.[51]

Positive airway pressure is the treatment of choice for sleep apnea; either continuous positive airway pressure for obstructive sleep apnea, or alternating pressures on inspiration and expiration for central sleep apnea. The pressurized air holds open the upper airway, much like a splint, and is delivered via an interface, which may take the form of a mask or nasal pillows. Care must be used in mask selection among patients with MS. For those with comorbid trigeminal neuralgia, certain masks may exacerbate facial pain. Another issue is how manual dexterity loss may also make it very difficult for patients with MS to use certain types of masks and fitting them properly to prevent air leaks.[52] Although positive airway pressure is the gold standard treatment for sleep apnea, custom fabricated dental appliances may be useful for patients who do not have the dexterity to manage positive airway pressure or who cannot tolerate it. Dental appliances work in obstructive sleep apnea by advancing the lower jaw forward and opening the upper airway.[53] These devices are effective in opening the airway, but again, in patients with MS with trigeminal neuralgia, they may exacerbate facial pain.[52]

RESTLESS LEG SYNDROME

Restless leg syndrome is characterized by a strong urge to move the legs and is often accompanied by uncomfortable sensations, such as pain and burning and tingling, among others.[54] The symptoms improve with movement and occur or become worse during the evening and night. Restless leg syndrome is observed commonly in patients with MS and worsens with both age and advancing disability. Restless leg syndrome severity is increased in patients with MS who experience comorbid restless leg syndrome, compared with those with the sole diagnosis of restless leg syndrome.[55] Patients with MS who experience restless leg syndrome have significant insomnia and poor sleep quality. They also tend to medicate more frequently with hypnotic and antidepressant medications.

There is no one test or procedure that will lead to the diagnosis of restless leg syndrome. A complete history and physical examination will be used to be rule out other common causes of restless leg syndrome, such as pregnancy, decreased serum iron, uremia, and sclerotic leg veins. A comprehensive medication history should be taken to determine if patients are taking medications that worsen restless leg syndrome, namely, antiemetics, antipsychotics, antidepressants, antihistamines, and dopamine antagonists.[40] Along with the history and complete physical examination, a full neurologic physical examination should be performed.

Four criteria are used to help establish the diagnosis of restless leg syndrome:

- Uncomfortable symptoms are associated with an urge to the move legs;
- Onset or worsening of urge to move the legs occurs during rest or inactivity;
- Partial or total relief of the urge to move or uncomfortable symptoms is achieved by movement or stretching; and
- Unpleasant symptoms or the urge to move occur during evening or night.[56]

Two measures have been shown to be helpful in determining the severity of restless leg syndrome among patients with MS. The International RLS Rating Scale is a self-reported, 10-item instrument (range, 0–40) that measures the severity of restless leg syndrome. Higher scores on this instrument indicate more severe restless leg syndrome symptoms.[57] The Expanded Disability Status Scale (EDSS) is an instrument administered by clinicians with a range of 0 (normal) to 10 (death). The EDSS cutpoint range of 4 to 6 usually is associated with the ability to ambulate. This instrument is commonly used and is internationally adopted as appropriate for use with patients with MS. Typically, patients with MS-associated restless leg syndrome also have higher scores on the EDSS, and thus experience greater disability than those with lower EDSS scores.[58]

The treatment of restless leg syndrome includes iron therapy, if indicated by laboratory results (serum iron level of <50). Medications used to treat the condition include dopamine agonists and alpha 2 ligands, such as gabapentin. It is important to note that use of dopamine agonists can lead to augmentation, which occurs when restless leg syndrome symptoms and signs occur at times during the day other than evening.[40]

NARCOLEPSY

Narcolepsy is a sleep disorder characterized by excessive daytime sleepiness; shortened sleep latency; early REM sleep onset; spontaneous bouts of daytime sleep with possible resulting difficulties in school, work, and driving performance; and fragmented nighttime sleep. It may also be associated with cataplexy, which is the sudden loss of voluntary muscle control, and nightmares at sleep onset or awakening.[59]

Narcolepsy is thought to be an autoimmune disorder associated with a decrease of hypocretin production in the hypothalamus. The disease is strongly associated with HLA, altered cytokines, and other immune system markers. MS may predispose patients to narcolepsy because of hypothalamic lesions or demyelination or through genetic predisposition. MS is closely associated with the HLA area located on the short arm of chromosome 6. Therefore, narcolepsy may or may not be associated with the development of MS and its subsequent course.[59]

The diagnosis of narcolepsy is initiated with a complete history and physical examination. A detailed medication history must be conducted to rule out sedating medications as a source of the signs and symptoms. Also, a complete sleep history, including completion of the Epworth Sleepiness Scale, should be taken to establish excessive daytime sleepiness.

Objective measures used to make the diagnosis of narcolepsy may include a 2-week period of sleep diary and actigraph monitoring to determine sleep and wake patterns. An overnight polysomnogram is essential to accurately determine if other sleep disorders are present and if patients have received adequate sleep before the gold standard test for narcolepsy: the Multiple Sleep Latency Test. On the morning immediately after the overnight polysomnogram, the Multiple Sleep Latency Test is conducted to determine mean sleep latency and the presence of sleep onset REM sleep. Patients take four to five 20-minute naps during which their sleep latencies and evidence of sleep onset REM episodes are monitored. Presence of a mean sleep latency of 8 minutes or less and REM sleep onset within the first 15 minutes of sleep are criteria for the diagnosis of narcolepsy.[60]

Treatment for narcolepsy includes the use of modafinil or methylphenidate and an antidepressant (to suppress REM sleep and decrease cataplexy symptoms). For patients with hypothalamic lesions, high doses of methylprednisone may be used. Nonpharmacologic treatment includes counseling and a structured sleep–wake schedule that includes daytime sleep.[61]

INSOMNIA

Insomnia, defined as a failure to initiate or maintain sleep, is a common concern of patients with MS.[62] Reported prevalence rates vary between just over 30% to 50%.[10,40,62] Insomnia may be present as a condition or as a symptom related to disease processes of or therapeutics used for MS. It is associated with depression,

Table 2
Instruments and diagnostics used to screen for conditions associated with sleep disturbance in MS

Instrument/Questionnaires	Instrument Description	Indication
Kurtze Expanded Disability Status Scale (EDSS)	A scale used to measure and quantify the disability status and level of functioning of people living with MS. The EDSS provides a total score on a scale that ranges from 0 to 10. The first levels 1.0–4.5 refer to people with a high degree of ambulatory ability and the subsequent levels 5.0–9.5 refer to the loss of ambulatory ability. The total EDSS score is determined by 2 factors: gait and FS scores.	Level of disability in MS
Kurtze Functional System Score (FSS)	The FSS is one-half of a 2-part system (the EDSS is other part of the system) evaluating the type and severity of neurologic impairment in MS and is based on neurologic examination of independent functions. Based on a standard neurologic examination, the 7 functional systems (plus "other") are rated. The FSS include pyramidal, cerebellar, brain stem, sensory, bowel and bladder, visual, cerebral (or mental), and other. These ratings are then used in conjunction with observations and information concerning gait and use of assistive devices to rate the EDSS. Each of the FSS is an ordinal clinical rating scale ranging from 0 to 5 or 6.	Level of disability in MS
STOP-BANG Questionnaire	Eight yes/no questions related to the risk factors for obstructive sleep apnea; questions include snoring, daytime tiredness, observed apneas, high blood pressure, body mass index (>35 kg/m²), age (≥50 y), neck circumference (>40 cm), and gender (male)	Obstructive sleep apnea
Berlin Sleep Apnea Questionnaire	This 10-item survey is divided into 3 categories, with category 1 addressing snoring, category 2 identifying EDS, and category 3 assessing current blood pressure and body mass index. To be classified as at high risk for sleep apnea, an individual must qualify for at least 2 categories. The Berlin Questionnaire has a high degree of sensitivity and specificity for predicting sleep apnea in individuals.	Obstructive sleep apnea

(continued on next page)

Table 2
(continued)

Instrument/Questionnaires	Instrument Description	Indication
Multiple Sleep Latency Test (MSLT)	The observation typically consists of 5 scheduled naps, each nap opportunity lasting 20 min, separated by 2-hour breaks. During each of the nap opportunities, a person lies in bed in a darkened, quiet room and tries to go to sleep. The time that it takes a person to fall asleep is called the sleep latency. The person is allowed to sleep for a maximum of 15 min during each opportunity. The person is awakened if he or she does wake up on their own. If the person does not fall asleep within 20 min, the nap trial will end. Sensors are placed on the person's head, face, and chin and used to determine if the person reaches REM sleep. A sleep expert will interpret the data and validate a sleep disorder such as narcolepsy.	Narcolepsy
Epworth Sleepiness Scale	Eight-item self –administered questionnaire assessing the patient's likelihood of falling asleep under 8 common scenarios. Likelihood is scored between 0 (never) and 3(high chance) with a total score of 24 A score >10 is indicative of excessive daytime sleepiness	Daytime Sleepiness
Pittsburg Sleep Quality Index (PSQI)	19 self-rated questions widely used for assessing sleep quality over the previous month; the questions are grouped into 7 subscales: sleep quality, sleep latency, sleep duration, sleep efficiency, sleep disturbance, use of sleep medication and daytime dysfunction; a score of 5 on the global score is indicative of being a "poor" sleep	General sleep quality
Fatigue Severity Scale (FSS)	Nine self-administered questions designed to rate the severity of fatigue symptoms in patients with MS, applying a Likert scale (1 [strongly disagree] to 7 [strongly agree]) Patients with a score of 36/64 or higher are found to be suffering from fatigue	Fatigue
Modified Fatigue Impact Scale (MFIS-5)	Twenty-one items derived from interviews with patients with MS concerning how fatigue impacts their live; it consists of 3 subscales: physical, cognitive and psychosocial functioning	Fatigue

Insomnia Severity Index	Seven questions that relate to the timing of individuals' potential insomnia and the extent to which insomnia affects their quality of life. Each question is graded on a scale of 0–4. A cumulative score 15 or greater indicated clinically significant insomnia	Insomnia
Restless Legs Syndrome-Diagnostic Index (RLS-DI)	Ten item diagnostic algorithm helpful for distinguishing between RLS and common MS symptoms and response to treatment	Restless leg syndrome
Restless Leg Syndrome Rating Scale	Ten-item self-rating questionnaire that can help predict severity of RLS symptoms and response to treatment; scoring mild (score 1–10); moderate (score 11–20), severe (score 31–40)	Restless leg syndrome

fatigue, and a decreased quality of life. Specifically, in patients with MS, insomnia may exacerbate chronic pain[27] and may negatively impact cognitive functioning.[63]

Assessing insomnia involves a complete history, including a comprehensive medication and sleep history, as well as the use of substances such as nicotine and caffeine, which are wake promoting. A physical examination may be indicated. There are many subjective instruments used to assess insomnia. Among the most commonly used are the Insomnia Severity Index and a daily sleep diary.

Management of insomnia is based on whether the insomnia is a primary condition or if it is secondary to comorbid conditions or treatment regimes. In the case of secondary insomnia, comorbid conditions or treatments must be considered. Making changes in the treatment or medication regime may be necessary to bring about improvement in insomnia and associated excessive daytime sleepiness. Principles of sleep hygiene should be stressed with patients and their families, with the implementation of sleep diaries or actigraphy before and after sleep hygiene instruction. The use of pharmacologic agents such as hypnotics and antihistamines should be avoided.[64] In the event that these measures are ineffective, cognitive behavioral therapy may be an appropriate approach.[65]

SUMMARY

Sleep disturbance and sleep disorders are more common in individuals with MS than in the general population. It is evident that sleep disturbance and sleep disorders negatively affect patients with MS and lead to cognitive function, depression, fatigue, and the exacerbation of physiologic pain, which ultimately leads to a decreased quality of life.[10,63,66] Yet, it is reported that sleep is not consistently addressed with patients with MS.[64] It is important to identify modifiable risks that may improve sleep quality and the overall health of the person who has MS.[35] A sleep history should be included in the initial assessment of the patient with MS, along with detailed medication and substance history. Using these data, along with MS-specific symptomology and MRI findings, will inform the need for additional sleep-specific screening and testing. Providers who have a high index of suspicion for sleep disorders should be familiar with and use the common screening instruments described in **Table 2**. Patients who screen positively for a potential sleep disorder should receive a timely referral and appointment with a sleep medicine provider. A thorough evaluation of sleep disturbance should be conducted periodically along with all the other MS symptoms that may influence sleep like depression, anxiety, fatigue, pain, and bowel and bladder disturbance. A multidisciplinary team approach should be used to manage and address MS symptoms that affect sleep quality. This practice will ensure that each person receives holistic care that will optimize his or her quality of life and cognitive functioning. Future research is needed at large MS centers to demonstrate the effect of implementing a program that will screen, identify, refer, and manage sleep disturbance on the quality of life of individuals with MS.

CLINICS CARE POINTS

- Evaluate and appropriately treat related symptoms that could be the primary cause of sleep disturbance in patients with MS.
- Initiate and periodically screen patients who have a suspected sleep disorder using validated assessment tools and instruments.
- Discuss the value of sleep hygiene and quality sleep with your patients at regular clinic visits.

- Review the medications used in the treatment of MS and related symptoms that may affect sleep quality and make appropriate adjustments to prescribed regimens.
- Implement sleep assessments and gather a comprehensive sleep history as a part of your routine evaluation of patients with MS.

DISCLOSURE

None.

ACKNOWLEDGMENTS

The authors would like to thank Rebecca Billings for her assistance with our literary search for this article.

REFERENCES

1. Brownlee WJ, Hardy TA, Fazekas F, et al. Diagnosis of multiple sclerosis: progress and challenges. Lancet 2017;389(10076):1336–46.
2. Chitnis T, Glanz B, Jaffin S, et al. Demographics of pediatric-onset multiple sclerosis in an MS center population from the Northeastern United States. Mult Scler 2009;15(5):627–31.
3. Waldman A, Ghezzi A, Bar-Or A, et al. Multiple sclerosis in children: an update on clinical diagnosis, therapeutic strategies, and research. Lancet Neurol 2014; 13(9):936–48.
4. Martinelli V, Rodegher M, Moiola L, et al. Late onset multiple sclerosis: clinical characteristics, prognostic factors and differential diagnosis. Neurol Sci 2004; 25(4):s350–5.
5. Wallin MT, Culpepper WJ, Campbell JD, et al. The prevalence of MS in the United States. A population-based estimate using health claims data. Neurology 2019; 92(10):e1029–40.
6. Tullman MJ. Overview of the epidemiology, diagnosis, and disease progression associated with multiple sclerosis. Am J Manag Care 2013;19(2 Suppl):S15–20.
7. Thompson AJ, Banwell BL, Barkhof F, et al. Diagnosis of multiple sclerosis: 2017 revisions of the McDonald criteria. Lancet Neurol 2018;17(2):162–73.
8. National MS Society. 2020. Disease Modifying Therapies for MS. Available at: http://www.nationalmssociety.org/nationalmssociety/media/msnationalfiles/brochures/brochure-the-ms-disease-modifying-medications.pdf. Accessed July 15, 2020.
9. Klineova S, Lublin FD. Clinical course of multiple sclerosis. Cold Spring Harbor Perspect Med 2018;8(9):a028928.
10. Bamer AM, Johnson KL, Amtmann D, et al. Prevalence of sleep problems in individuals with multiple sclerosis. Mult Scler 2008;14(8):1127–30.
11. Merlino G, Fratticci L, Lenchig C, et al. Prevalence of 'poor sleep' among patients with multiple sclerosis: an independent predictor of mental and physical status. Sleep Med 2009;10(1):26–34.
12. Foschi M, Rizzo G, Liguori R, et al. Sleep-related disorders and their relationship with MRI findings in multiple sclerosis. Sleep Med 2019;56:90–7.
13. Oka Y, Kanbayashi T, Mezaki T, et al. Low CSF hypocretin-1/orexin-A associated with hypersomnia secondary to hypothalamic lesion in a case of multiple sclerosis. J Neurol 2004;251(7):885–6.

14. Nishino S, Kanbayashi T. Symptomatic narcolepsy, cataplexy and hypersomnia, and their implications in the hypothalamic hypocretin/orexin system. Sleep Med Rev 2005;9(4):269–310.

15. Zielinski MR, Systrom DM, Rose NR. Fatigue, sleep, and autoimmune and related disorders. Front Immunol 2019;10:1827.

16. Melamud L, Golan D, Luboshitzky R, et al. Melatonin dysregulation, sleep disturbances and fatigue in multiple sclerosis. J Neurol Sci 2012;314(1–2):37–40.

17. Pokryszko-Dragan A, Bilińska M, Gruszka E, et al. Sleep disturbances in patients with multiple sclerosis. Neurol Sci 2013;34(8):1291–6.

18. Attarian H, Applebee G, Applebee A, et al. Effect of eszopiclone on sleep disturbances and daytime fatigue in multiple sclerosis patients. Int J MS Care 2011; 13(2):84–90.

19. Kaminska M, Kimoff RJ, Benedetti A, et al. Obstructive sleep apnea is associated with fatigue in multiple sclerosis. Mult Scler 2012;18(8):1159–69.

20. Veauthier C. Sleep disorders in multiple sclerosis. Review. Curr Neurol Neurosci Rep 2015;15(5):21.

21. Tachibana N, Howard RS, Hirsch NP, et al. Sleep problems in multiple sclerosis. Eur Neurol 1994;34(6):320–32.

22. National MS Society. 2020. Symptom Management. Available at: https://www.nationalmssociety.org/For-Professionals/Clinical-Care/Managing-MS/Symptom-Management. Assessed October 22, 2020.

23. Veauthier C, Paul F. Sleep disorders in multiple sclerosis and their relationship to fatigue. Sleep Med 2014;15(1):5–14.

24. Brass SD, Duquette P, Proulx-Therrien J, et al. Sleep disorders in patients with multiple sclerosis. Sleep Med Rev 2010;14(2):121–9.

25. O'Connor AB, Schwid SR, Herrmann DN, et al. Pain associated with multiple sclerosis: systematic review and proposed classification. Pain 2008;137(1):96–111.

26. Schutte-Rodin S, Broch L, Buysse D, et al. Clinical guideline for the evaluation and management of chronic insomnia in adults. J Clin Sleep Med 2008;4(5): 487–504.

27. Tabrizi FM, Radfar M. Fatigue, sleep quality, and disability in relation to quality of life in multiple sclerosis. Int J MS Care 2015;17(6):268–74.

28. Simmons RD, Tribe KL, McDonald EA. Living with multiple sclerosis: longitudinal changes in employment and the importance of symptom management. J Neurol 2010;257(6):926–36.

29. Krupp L. Fatigue is intrinsic to multiple sclerosis (MS) and is the most commonly reported symptom of the disease. Mult Scler 2006;12(4):367–8.

30. Bakshi R. Fatigue associated with multiple sclerosis: diagnosis, impact and management. Mult Scler 2003;9(3):219–27.

31. National MS Society (2009). Students with MS & the academic setting: a handbook for school personnel. Available at: National MS Society. 2020. Symptom Management. Available at: https://www.nationalmssociety.org/For-Professionals/Clinical-Care/Managing-MS/Symptom-Management. Accessed October 20, 2020.

32. DeLuca J. Fatigue: its definition, its study and its future. In: Deluca J, editor. Fatigue as a Window to the brain. Cambridge: The MIT Press; 2005. p. 1–10.

33. Caminero A, Bartolomé M. Sleep disturbances in multiple sclerosis. J Neurol Sci 2011;309(1–2):86–91.

34. Čarnická Z, Kollár B, Šiarnik P, et al. Sleep disorders in patients with multiple sclerosis. J Clin Sleep Med 2015;11(5):553–7.

35. Bøe Lunde HM, Aae TF, Indrevåg W, et al. Poor sleep in patients with multiple sclerosis. PLoS One 2012;7(11):e49996.

36. Milto L. Sleep Tight. Momentum-The Magazine and Blog of the National MS Society. 2019. Available at: https://momentummagazineonline.com/sleep-tight/. Accessed October 08, 2020.

37. Mendozzi L, Tronci F, Garegnani M, et al. Sleep disturbance and fatigue in mild relapsing remitting multiple sclerosis patients on chronic immunomodulant therapy: an actigraphic study. Mult Scler 2010;16(2):238–47.

38. Nadjar Y, Coutelas E, Prouteau P, et al. Injection of interferon-beta in the morning decreases flu-like syndrome in many patients with multiple sclerosis. Clin Neurol Neurosurg 2011;113(4):316–22.

39. Hughes AJ, Parmenter BA, Haselkorn JK, et al. Sleep and its associations with perceived and objective cognitive impairment in individuals with multiple sclerosis. J Sleep Res 2017;26(4):428–35.

40. Braley TJ, Boudreau EA. Sleep Disorders in Multiple Sclerosis. Curr Neurol Neurosci Rep 2016;16(5):50.

41. Horner RL. Pathophysiology of objective sleep apnea. J Cardiopulm Rehabil Prev 2008;28(5):289–98.

42. Johns M. Rethinking the assessment of sleepiness. Sleep Med Rev 1998; 2(1):3–15.

43. Chiu HY, Chen PY, Chuang LP, et al. Diagnostic accuracy of the Berlin questionnaire, STOP-BANG, STOP, and Epworth sleepiness scale in detecting obstructive sleep apnea: a bivariate meta-analysis. Sleep Med Rev 2017;36:57–70.

44. Kapur VK, Auckley DH, Chowdhuri S, et al. Clinical practice guideline for diagnostic testing for adult obstructive sleep apnea: an American Academy of Sleep Medicine clinical practice guideline. J Clin Sleep Med 2017;13(03):479–504.

45. Hensen HA, Krishnan AV, Eckert DJ. Sleep-disordered breathing in people with multiple sclerosis: prevalence, pathophysiological mechanisms, and disease consequences. Front Neurol 2018;8:740.

46. Kallweit U, Baumann CR, Harzheim M, et al. Fatigue and sleep-disordered breathing in multiple sclerosis: a clinically relevant association? Mult Scler Int 2013;2013:286581.

47. Rundo JV. Obstructive sleep apnea basics. Cleve Clin J Med 2019;86(9 Suppl 1):2–9.

48. Learmonth YC, Dlugonski D, Pilutti LA, et al. Psychometric properties of the Fatigue Severity Scale and the Modified Fatigue Impact Scale. J Neurol Sci 2013; 331(1–2):102–7.

49. Chung F, Abdullah HR, Liao P. STOP-bang questionnaire: a practical approach to screen for obstructive sleep apnea. Chest 2016;149(3):631–8.

50. Donovan LM, Kapur VK. Prevalence and characteristics of central compared to obstructive sleep apnea: analyses from the sleep heart health study cohort. Sleep 2016;39(7):1353–9.

51. National Multiple Sclerosis Society and Multiple Sclerosis Society of Canada. Managing pain and sleep in multiple sclerosis. 2012. Available at: https://mssociety.ca/en/pdf/managing-pain-and-sleep-issues-in-ms-EN.pdf. Accessed October 1, 2020.

52. Braley TJ. Overview: a framework for the discussion of sleep in multiple sclerosis. Curr Sleep Med Rep 2017;3(4):263–71.

53. Sakkas GK, Giannaki CD, Karatzaferi C, et al. Sleep abnormalities in multiple sclerosis. Curr Treat Options Neurol 2019;21(1):4.

54. Li Y, Munger KL, Batool-Anwar S, et al. Association of multiple sclerosis with restless legs syndrome and other sleep disorders in women. Neurology 2012;78(19): 1500–6.
55. Manconi M, Ferini-Strambi L, Filippi M, et al. Multicenter case-control study on restless legs syndrome in multiple sclerosis: the REMS study. Sleep 2008; 31(7):944–52.
56. Bayard M, Avonda T, Wadzinski J. Restless legs syndrome. Am Fam Physician 2008;78(2):235–40.
57. Sharon D, Allen RP, Martinez-Martin P, et al. Validation of the self-administered version of the international Restless Legs Syndrome study group severity rating scale - The sIRLS. Sleep Med 2019;54:94–100.
58. Cohen JA, Reingold SC, Polman CH, et al. Disability outcome measures in multiple sclerosis clinical trials: current status and future prospects. Lancet Neurol 2012;11(5):467–76.
59. Martinez-Orozco FJ, Vicario JL, De Andres C, et al. Comorbidity of narcolepsy type 1 with autoimmune diseases and other immunopathological disorders: a case-control study. J Clin Med Res 2016;8(7):495–505.
60. Schneider L, Mignot E. Diagnosis and management of narcolepsy. Semin Neurol 2017;37(4):446–60.
61. Lunde HM, Bjorvatn B, Myhr KM, et al. Clinical assessment and management of sleep disorders in multiple sclerosis: a literature review. Acta Neurol Scand Suppl 2013;196:24–30.
62. Brass SD, Li CS, Auerbach S. The underdiagnosis of sleep disorders in patients with multiple sclerosis. J Clin Sleep Med 2014;10(9):1025–31.
63. van Geest Q, Westerik B, van der Werf YD, et al. The role of sleep on cognition and functional connectivity in patients with multiple sclerosis. J Neurol 2017; 264(1):72–80.
64. Braley TJ, Segal BM, Chervin RD. Underrecognition of sleep disorders in patients with multiple sclerosis. J Clin Sleep Med 2015;11(1):81.
65. Siengsukon CF, Alshehri M, Williams C, et al. Feasibility and treatment effect of cognitive behavioral therapy for insomnia in individuals with multiple sclerosis: a pilot randomized controlled trial. Mult Scler Relat Disord 2020;40:101958.
66. Amtmann D, Askew RL, Kim J, et al. Pain affects depression through anxiety, fatigue, and sleep in multiple sclerosis. Rehabil Psychol 2015;60(1):81–90.

Sleep-Wake Disturbances in Oncology

Kristi A. Acker, DNP, PhD, FNP-BC, AOCNP, ACHPN[a],*, Patricia Carter, PhD, RN, CNS[b]

KEYWORDS

- Sleep disturbance • Insomnia • Cancer • Oncology • Cancer fatigue
- Insomnia management

KEY POINTS

- Sleep disturbance commonly occurs in oncology settings.
- Many factors influence whether or not sleep issues are assessed in clinical oncology practice.
- Sleep assessment requires a conscientious, detailed, and multifaceted assessment skillset.

BACKGROUND

Sleep disturbance, dyssomnia, circadian rhythm disorder, insomnia, and sleep-wake cycle change; many terms, yet few absolute single solutions for successful management. Sleep-wake disturbance, including poor quality of sleep, is a common occurrence observed in patients with cancer.[1–3] Insomnia, is considered one of the most common sleep-wake disorders reported in patients with cancer.[2,3] For many oncology patients, sleep-wake changes, including insomnia, are situational and resolve without the need for intervention. However, evidence suggests that mismanagement of sleep-wake disturbances can lead to chronic insomnia, ultimately resulting in a decreased quality of life, increased relationship strain, compromised immunity, and work interruptions.[2,4] Evaluating sleep-wake disturbance in oncology settings requires a conscientious, detailed, and multifaceted assessment skillset to better understand the complexities, and often emotionally laden, patient and caregiver distress unique to oncology. Many factors result in apathetic assessment of sleep-wake disturbances in oncology patients, which include competing symptom burden, patient reluctance to self-report sleep-wake changes, and provider time constraints, inconsistent assessment, among others. Integrating a screening tool into practice can help provide a timely sleep assessment and allow for continuous monitoring for therapeutic management.[5] This article provides a brief overview of sleep-wake disturbance in patients

a Capstone College of Nursing, University of Alabama, Office 3029, Box 870358, Tuscaloosa, AL 35487, USA; b Capstone College of Nursing, University of Alabama, 3012 Nursing, Box 870358, Tuscaloosa, AL 35487, USA
* Corresponding author.
E-mail address: kaacker@ua.edu

Nurs Clin N Am 56 (2021) 175–187
https://doi.org/10.1016/j.cnur.2021.03.001
0029-6465/21/© 2021 Elsevier Inc. All rights reserved.
nursing.theclinics.com

with cancer, including the unique need for a multifaceted provider assessment. Common management strategies, special considerations, and novel therapies are discussed.

DEFINING INSOMNIA

Due to inconsistent terminology, and overlapping symptomology, sleep-wake disturbances are underrecognized in oncology settings. The lack of recognition further complicates proper assessment and treatment thereof. Insomnia is one of the most commonly noted sleep-wake disturbance encountered in oncology. Insomnia, which can be either acute or chronic in nature can be one of the most challenging, most unrecognized, and most undertreated symptom burdens in oncology. Insomnia is a condition that can result in cognitive decline and decreased social engagement, which may have far-reaching consequences that can negatively impact disease outcome. Insomnia is best described as sleep interruption, difficulty initiating and/or maintaining sleep, or early awakenings despite adequate opportunity for sleep. If not appropriately addressed, insomnia may well extend beyond active treatment and negatively impact oncology patient survivorship, especially as it relates to quality of life. Insomnia is also a main contributor to cancer fatigue, which is a widely recognized phenomena in oncology settings.

PREVALENCE

Quantifying the prevalence of sleep-wake disturbances in oncology often proves challenging. Many comorbid conditions, in which insomnia can fall into the "cluster" of symptoms are more frequently seen in oncology settings in comparison to the general population. Predisposing factors for prevalence of sleep-wake disturbances; specifically, insomnia, is age, female gender, and those with a personal or family history of insomnia, depression, and anxiety.[1] According to the National Cancer Institute,[6] additional risks factors can include opioids, antidepressants, dietary supplements, physical and/or psychological stress, delirium and daytime seizures, snoring, and headaches. Insomnia can occur at any age and affects 10% to 50% of the adult population,[7] with an even much higher occurrence in oncology settings.[3,8]

SLEEP IN ONCOLOGY

It is not uncommon for oncology patients to have greater anxiety and depression compared with the general population. Patients and providers alike anticipate sleep disturbances will occur at some point along the disease trajectory; but interestingly, consistent assessment for identifying sleep disturbances is not widely integrated into oncology practice. Sleep-wake disturbances may emerge based on intrinsic (eg, familiar history, aging) and/or extrinsic factors (eg, adverse effects of medications, disease burden). Just the physical presence of the patient in an oncology setting can result in angst and unrest. There are a number of stressful factors that accompany oncology patients. It is not uncommon that with an initial diagnosis, patients have often experienced weeks, if not months, of burdensome symptoms, abnormal radiological reports, biopsy attempt(s), and numerous related medical clinic visits. Further, the influence of lived experiences, has a potential for adding yet another complex layer of emotions that can impact sleep-wake disturbances, especially with a new cancer diagnosis. Even temporary extrinsic causes of sleep-wake disturbances can have long-term impact on sleep hygiene. One of the first steps to help identify and manage sleep-wake disturbance begins with provider awareness, and an understanding of current guidelines for managing sleep. Evidence supports that unrecognized and undertreated sleep-wake disorders could ultimately result in chronic problems with insomnia.

SYMPTOM OVERLAP

Adding to the complexities of the disorder is a constellation of overlapping symptoms that can exist despite different diagnoses (ie, pain and depression). In fact, "clusters" of psychological symptoms have been found in patients with cancer including high levels of anxiety, depression, insomnia, and cognitive impairments.[9] Cancer fatigue, which is a common phenomenon in oncology, can result in daytime sleeping patterns that can impact quality nocturnal sleep cycles. Providers are urged to use a multidimensional approach in exploring sleep-wake disturbances to assess underlying etiologies such as pain, depression, pulmonary disease, substance abuse, hormonal secretion imbalances, or paraneoplastic syndromes, among others. Identifying an underlying condition(s) is of utmost importance to simultaneously manage sleep-wake disturbance in a sustainable and successful manner. Sleep-wake disturbances can be complicated by a plethora of comorbidities, such as obstructive sleep apnea and restless legs syndrome, which are 2 common conditions encountered in oncology settings. **Fig. 1** depicts the various factors that can inhibit and adversely impact quality sleep patterns in patients with cancer.

Varying types of cancer stages in treatment modalities influence sleep-wake patterns. For example, women who are diagnosed with breast cancer may have issues maintaining quality sleep patterns due to hormonal imbalances that can lead to menopausal symptoms such as hot flashes and night sweats. Savard and colleagues[10] noted that women (diagnosed with breast or other gynecologic malignancy) who have prechemotherapy insomnia were potentially more vulnerable to immune alterations and chemotherapy-associated infection rates. Stone and colleagues[11] explored cancer-specific mortality and all-cause mortality among survivors of cancer and found that both short and long sleep durations are associated with an increased risk of cancer-specific mortality.

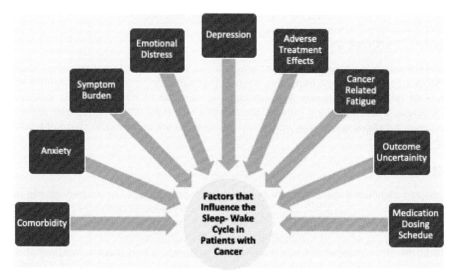

Fig. 1. Influences on sleep-wake disturbance in oncology.[1,10]

ANTINEOPLASTIC THERAPY

In addition, specific antineoplastic treatment modalities may use high-dose cortico-steroids that can inhibit sleep (eg, bortezomib, lenalidomide, and dexamethasone [VRD] and cyclophosphamide, doxorubicin, vincristine, and prednisone [CHOP]). Corticosteroids are frequently used to prevent allergic reactions, control nausea and vomiting, increase appetite, reduce inflammation, and for a multitude of palliation of burdensome effects of advanced cancer.

CORONAVIRUS DISEASE 2019 IMPACT ON SLEEP

Coronavirus disease 2019 (COVID-19) should also be accounted for during oncology psychosocial assessment. As our nation faces challenges surrounding COVID-19 and social distancing, patients who are newly diagnosed are separated from family/friend support systems, due to visiting restrictions deployed in most medical facilities. It is often the caregivers who provide support and help minimize the anxiety surrounding oncology clinic visits. In short, receiving a cancer diagnosis is overwhelming and stressful, and having adequate support is necessary in oncology settings.

CANCER, AGE, AND SLEEP

The risk of cancer increases with age, as does the risk for comorbidity. The geriatric population has a higher propensity to have multiple chronic conditions, making them at a higher risk for sleep-wake disturbances, specifically insomnia. Insomnia is commonly seen in patients with pulmonary, chromic pain, heart failure, substance abuse disorders, among other comorbid conditions. Cancer often develops in addition to these conditions, which further compounds the complexities for appropriate assessment and management. With normal aging, sleep changes occur that reduce sleep quality. Unfortunately, the likelihood of chronic sleep-wake changes is greater in the geriatric population, and special caution must be made when considering adverse effects. Providers must start at the lowest possible dose and monitor more frequently when introducing pharmacologic treatment modalities. Other considerations in the geriatric population include underlying symptoms of dementia including, but not limited to increased fall risks, sundowning, and delirium.

PATIENT-CAREGIVER DYAD

Little is known about the patient and caregiver dyad as it relates to patient sleep-wake disturbances in oncology. Early data support that caregivers do suffer the negative effects of patient sleep-wake disturbances (eg, decreased mood, anxiety, daytime sleepiness, irritably, among others). Sleep-wake disturbances can adversely impact caregiver functioning and may contribute to missed work and overutilization of health care resources.

ASSESSMENT

Although significant gaps remain in sleep-wake assessment, dedicated efforts to improve provider awareness of the benefits of quality sleep in oncology can result in meaningful practice change. For example, advancements in pain evaluation (which is commonly reported in symptom dyads) has become commonplace in oncology. Moreover, pain assessment has evolved into a standard and pivotal component of oncology care planning. In fact, evaluating pain has become so routine that quantitative pain assessment is commonly referred to as the fifth vital sign. With the high prevalence of sleep-wake disturbances forecasted and observed in patients with cancer, why then is sleep assessment not a priority as well in oncology settings? Research provided a rich foundation for linking pain to patient outcomes, which incentivized oncology providers to adequately manage painful symptom burden. Just as progress was made concerning physical pain management in oncology, providers must familiarize themselves as to the impact of sleep-wake disturbances on overall patient outcomes. The variations for sleep intake screening may result in patient underreport due to the intense focus on the cancer diagnosis.

Numerous systematic reviews have been recently published that identify and evaluate the effectiveness of sleep therapies in cancer populations.[12–16] Universally, the recommendation is that all patients with cancer should be assessed for the presence of sleep-wake disruptions. Common sleep disorders in persons with cancer include insomnia and excessive daytime sleepiness (EDS). The initial screening assessment for these common disorders can simply begin by asking patients 3 questions:

- Are you having problems falling asleep?
- Are you having problems staying asleep?
- Are you experiencing overwhelming sleepiness?

If the answer is "yes" to any of these questions, the next step is a focused assessment of the nature of the sleep disturbance, contributing factors, and daytime consequences. The validity and reliability have been established for a number of sleep disorder assessment tools. However, many are not "clinic friendly," meaning that administration and/or scoring may be time-consuming and/or difficult. Given the environmental pressure to be as efficient as possible in the clinical setting, assessment tools must be valid and reliable as well as practical. We recommend the use of the following instruments in the clinical setting.

- Insomnia can be reliably assessed with the Insomnia Severity Index (ISI).[17] This 7-item scale assesses the level of classic sleep symptoms and daytime disruptions. The ISI is quickly administered and easily scored into 4 categories: 0 to 7 = no clinical insomnia, 8 to 14 = subthreshold insomnia (mild), 15 to 21 = clinical insomnia (moderate severity), and 22 to 28 = severe insomnia.
- Sleep quality can be assesses using the Pittsburgh Sleep Quality Index developed by Buysse and colleagues.[18] Using this self-rated questionnaire, 7 component scores, including sleep quality, sleep latency, sleep duration, habitual sleep efficiency, sleep disturbances, use of sleep aids, and daytime dysfunction, are assessed. One global score is calculated, with 0 being the best score versus 21 the worst. Scores ≤5 are associated with good sleep and greater than 5 are associated with poor sleep quality.
- EDS can be screened quickly using the Epworth Sleepiness Scale.[19] This 8-item scale assesses the likelihood of an individual falling asleep in a variety of situations (eg, riding in a car, watching TV, talking with someone). Scores range from 0 to 24 with higher scores indicating more sleepiness. Results fall into 3 categories: 0 to 10 = Normal (no EDS), 11 to 16 = EDS, and greater than 16 = High EDS.
- Self-reported sleep logs and/or diaries have shown to add value in assessing sleep in all settings. A multitude of sleep templates can be electronically accessed, or patients can self-record awakenings, sleep duration, and sleep efficiency over a 2-week time interval. Having a record of the sleeping patterns can help guide the provider as to the severity of the sleep-wake changes and the potential negative impact on quality of life.

MANAGEMENT

Correlations in symptomatology in oncology settings are commonly reported. Over the past decade there has been an emphasis on management of cancer-related fatigue (in which insomnia can worsen the symptom burden). As with many aspects of oncology treatment, managing adverse effects, such as fatigue, remains in constant motion. The use of common hematopoietic interventions for treating cancer-related fatigue have been amended.[20] Therefore, oncology providers must remain current regarding best practice for managing sleep-wake disturbances. Various treatment approaches exist and aggressive attempts for identifying and properly managing underlying etiologies (ie, metabolic and neuroendocrine disruptions) should be a priority. Further patient and caregiver education remain a necessary goal. Developing oncology care planning must remain patient centered and requires frequent goal discussions, and often an interdisciplinary approach for best management.[21,22]

In oncology, the mainstay in management practices centers initially on nonpharmacologic interventions, including cognitive behavioral therapy (CBT) strategies that have shown to be successful in patients with cancer.[23] Individualized and combined nonpharmacologic interventions should be first-line treatment, especially with the potential for adverse effects and drug to drug interactions with the addition of pharmacologic modalities. However, benefits for combining medication with nonpharmacologic strategies are recognized for managing challenging sleep-wake disturbances. Managing sleep-wake disorders is not uniform and conflicting data exist as to the benefit superiority of nonphonological measures over pharmacologic intervention.[2,24,25] One constant found in the evidence is that maladaptive patient responses can lead to chronic issues with sleep-wake disturbances, such as chronic insomnia, if sleep-wake disturbances are not assessed and managed in patients with cancer.[3] **Table 1** provides a brief overview of best practice strategies for managing sleep-wake disturbances in oncology settings.

It is critical that the oncology provider understand the natural sleep pattern and assess for influences (specific to oncology) that can interfere with quality sleep. The integration of sleep management strategies should ideally be integrated into existing oncology screening and management practices. Cognitive behavioral interventions, including mindfulness-based stress reduction has been shown to be important as first-line treatment.[23] Lifestyle modifications should also be integrated into the care plan. If the oncology provider suspects possible sleep apnea as the origin of the sleep-wake disturbance, the referral for a more comprehensive sleep analysis may be warranted. Evidence has demonstrated that treatment with positive airway pressure (continuous positive airway pressure, bilevel positive airway pressure) can improve the quality of sleep. In addition, patients may benefit from other interventions such as the utilization of oral appliances.

In general, the sleep-wake rhythms of all patients can be supported through education regarding healthy sleep habits. Educational materials are provided by a number of reliable sources (eg, American Cancer Society, National Cancer Institute) that can be downloaded and provided to patients. Although these materials are helpful and provide general recommendations, it is important to include as part of the treatment plan an ongoing assessment of sleep disruptions that may exacerbated by cancer therapies (eg, steroids, endocrine therapy, stimulants, among others). Patients need to be informed that their sleep is likely to disrupted, but they need to communicate with their cancer care team to receive support to minimize disruptions. As we have discussed previously, a robust sleep-wake cycle positively influences morbidity and mortality of the patient with cancer.

Table 1 Multimodality approach to sleep-wake disorder in oncology	
Aggressive Symptom Management	**Managing Nausea, Vomiting, Hiccups, Cough, Dyspnea, and so forth**
Nonpharmacologic interventions[26,27]	*Cognitive Behavioral Therapy (CBT):* (ie, mindfulness training; relaxation techniques + biofeedback: muscle relaxation, abdominal breathing, mental focusing/imagery; sleep education and hygiene training) • *Environmental control:* (ie, temperature controlled (cool), dim lighting, background white noise, technology limits, comfortable mattress, minimize scheduled sleep interruptions) • *Lifestyle modifications:* (ie, increase daytime activity/ exercise; limit daytime sleeping; keep a sleep routine even on weekends; small evening meal, limiting fluids before bedtime including caffeine; increase daylight exposure; avoid nighttime nicotine; use bed only for sleep and sex; get out of bed if you cannot fall asleep within 20 min) Centers for Disease Control and Prevention and American Academy of Sleep Medicine
Treatment of underlying etiology	Initiation of palliative radiation and/or systemic antineoplastic therapies; initiating pain medication regimens and treating "total pain" including psychosocial/spiritual distress; treating underlying endocrine issues; reducing stimulating agents such as corticosteroids; treating substance abuse disorders
*Pharmacologic interventions[27]	*Short-intermediate acting benzodiazepine receptor agonists* (ie, zolpidem, zaleplon, temazepam, eszopiclone) or *Melatonin receptor agonists* (ramelteon) or *Orexin receptor agonist* (suvorexant) *Sedating antidepressants* (ie, mirtazapine; doxepin; trazodone; amitriptyline) *Neuroleptics* (ie, gabapentin; tiagabine) *Over the counter* (ie, melatonin, valerian; diphenhydramine) *Refer to the American Academy of Sleep Medicine Clinical Practice Guideline for comprehensive recommendations*
Complementary therapies	Acupuncture; Forest therapy; Benson's relaxation response; complementary environment approaches; acupoint

Careful consideration of the mechanisms of action and potential interactions with cancer therapies must be kept in mind and potential risks may outweigh the benefits associated with these medications.

Pharmacotherapy for insomnia and obstructive sleep apnea have shown mixed results and given the potential for interaction with cancer therapies, they are not recommended.

CANCER–SLEEP INTERACTION

It is difficult to fully explain the cause and effect in cancer-associated sleep disruption. Differences in cancer types, treatment regimens, and patient behaviors and characteristics makes the underlying mechanisms unclear. Cancer seems to disrupt sleep, and poor sleep promotes tumorigenesis and cancer progression[28] and has been shown to increase risk of cancer mortality up to 17%.[29] Furthermore, poor sleep is associated with reduced patient quality of life even when controlling for multiple factors like metastasis, age, cortisol concentrations, estrogen receptor expression, and comorbid depression.[30]

NOVEL INTERVENTIONS

Forest therapy: The natural environment can be used as a therapeutic resource for emotional relaxation and stress management for people who live in cities. Kim and colleagues[31] found that total sleep time increased by 30 minutes on average and sleep efficiency increased by 8% following 6 days of forest therapy.

Benson's relaxation response is a focused relaxation method that Harorani and colleagues[32] used in a clinical trial that resulted in significant 24-hour and 48-hour improvement in self-reported sleep quality as compared with control (standard care).

Melatonin is a hormone chemically related to serotonin that is produced by the pineal gland in the midbrain and plays a key role in circadian rhythmicity. Kurdi and Muthukalai[33] found promising improvements in insomnia symptoms in a double-blind study of 3 mg of melatonin administered 2 hours before bedtime compared with placebo.

Complementary environment approaches: Creating a sleep-promoting environment is an important element in good sleep hygiene. Some small studies have reported positive results on sleep quality in patients with cancer through the use of aromatherapy,[34] bright light,[35] or music.[36]

Acupoint stimulation includes both acupuncture and acupressure techniques to stimulate specific points and restore balance (Qi). Liu and colleagues[37] found some support for the use of these techniques to improve sleep quality in patients with cancer; however, the findings are limited due to the small number of clinical trials that have been performed.

SUMMARY AND FUTURE DIRECTIONS

Sleep is a basic necessity for health and well-being across species, yet it can be easily disrupted, resulting in potentially devastating health outcomes. Cancer from onset through diagnosis, therapy, and survivorship is a complex and disruptive force. This disruptive force often wreaks havoc on the sleep-wake cycle of the individual who is diagnosed. However, all is not lost. As we have explored in this article, there is strong empirical evidence of the importance of assessing for sleep-wake disturbances in persons with cancer and effective therapies to improve sleep quality. It is important to acknowledge the gaps that persist between the empirically supported assessment and therapeutics and the practical applicability to clinical practice. Translational work is needed to bridge these gaps and to provide realistic assessment and therapeutic approaches that can be used in community oncology practices. In addition, work is needed to support the return on investment for clinical practice to implement these approaches. It is only when we are able to clearly demonstrate a financial return on investment for practices that we will obtain buy-in for wide application of these therapies.

CASE STUDY

SJ is a 51-year-old woman who was recently diagnosed with a Stage 3a ER+/PR+, Her2(−) infiltrating ductal carcinoma of the right breast. Family history reveals that her maternal grandmother died of ovarian cancer (age 72) and that SJ's biological sister was recently diagnosed with Stage 4 breast cancer (age 49). Immediately after receiving her pathology report and postsurgical follow-up, SJ was provided information regarding the need for medical oncology consultation; although SJ was reminded that only 1 person could accompany her to the oncology clinic due to COVID-19 visitation restrictions.

Two Weeks Later...

SJ and her daughter present to her initial oncology consultative appointment. SJ was found to have a high genomic test score and adjuvant chemotherapy with dose-dense doxorubicin/cyclophosphamide/paclitaxel and endocrine therapy was recommended. SJ was also provided a referral to the radiation oncology clinic to discuss options for treatment. The treatment plan was discussed in detail by the medical oncologists, as were the potential adverse effects of therapy.

1. Identify 3 situational stressors that SJ is likely experiencing that could negatively impact her sleep-wake cycle?
2. Discuss hormonal changes that would potentially impact SJ's sleep cycle?
3. Identify 3 potential antineoplastic treatment related side effects that commonly affect the sleep-wake cycle?

CASE STUDY DISCUSSION

Question 1: There are several situational stressors that SJ will likely experience. First, the stressor of having a new diagnosis of breast cancer. This factor alone can result in situational stress that can directly impact her sleep and ability to maintain quality sleep. Even the task of communicating her new diagnosis to family/friends can cause emotional distress and anxiety, not to mention, the body image adjustments that SJ will experience following surgery. In addition, SJ has a lived experience that she is bringing to the table. Her grandmother died of ovarian cancer, and her biological sister was diagnosed with metastatic breast cancer. It is unlikely that a provider would know details about SJ's lived experiences with cancer, although SJ's family history and lived experiences has the potential to negatively impact her perception of the new cancer diagnosis. Finally, the uncertainty concerning the outcome of her diagnosis, and her upcoming medical oncology visits/treatment regimen are situational stressors.

Question 2: This question poses some of the most complex issues that patients deal with regarding malignancy, especially women diagnosed with breast cancer. SJ is 51 years of age and from the information provided there is no indication as to whether or not she is premenopausal, perimenopausal, or postmenopausal. SJ could potentially be on hormone replacement therapy at the time of diagnosis, which would be discontinued due to her new ER+ breast cancer. Any sudden change in hormonal balance, can result in profound menopausal symptoms (eg, hot flashes and night sweats). Further, based on her own family history, SJ is likely to receive information for genetic testing. Should SJ have BRCA gene mutation, SJ will be making decisions for undergoing prophylactic oophorectomy, which would have a direct impact on hormonal changes. Chemotherapy alone will be a significant factor resulting in menopausal changes if she is premenopausal entering into treatment. The long-term impact on endocrine treatment plan can result in menopausal symptoms, such as such as frequent hot flashes and night sweats, which may in turn disrupt sleep patterns and emotional fluctuations, along with other potential adverse effects such as joint pain.

Question 3: Identifying side effects of chemotherapy that can impact quality sleep can be complex. SJ will be undergoing doxorubicin-based chemotherapy as well as treatment with a taxane. Doxorubicin-based therapies are considered highly emetic; therefore, close observation and frequent toxicity checks will be indicated. In addition, the impact of doxorubicin-based therapy contributes to hormone imbalances, especially for women who are premenopausal before treatment. Based on the potential risk for neuropathy and the discomfort and pain that could potentially result, interferences with sleep should be assessed often, due the potential for chronic symptoms that negatively impact quality of life and late-term side effects of therapy. In addition to the chemotherapeutic variables that have a direct influence on sleep, the use of corticosteroids often given for their center synergistic impact on anti-emetic prophylaxis can also resort in varying degrees sleep-wake disturbances.

Case summary: Acute and potentially long-term distress can result following a cancer diagnosis. Many of the acute factors for sleep-wake disturbances in oncology settings can be managed; however, long-term consequences can occur due to undiagnosed and/or undermanaged sleep-wake disturbances. With careful system assessment and an aggressive approach in managing comorbid symptom burden(s), most sleep-wake disturbances are expected to resolve with the implementation of nonpharmacologic ± short-term pharmacologic interventions. Understanding that a coexisting medical disorder can result in additional distress, and that cancer diagnosis and treatments can result in a heightened environmental arousal, increased symptom burden (eg, fatigue, emotional distress, depression, fatigue, and excessive worry about the future outcomes), the oncology provider should encourage SJ to self-manage with identification of the problem and provide education and training regarding nonpharmacologic strategies. The oncology provider should also consider short-term pharmacologic intervention and use sleep specialist referral for complicated sleep-wake disturbances that are not responsive to initial treatment. Also, the oncology provider should assess for underlying pulmonary condition(s) and consider prompt referral allowing for detailed sleep analyses. It is highly recommended that oncology providers become familiar with the range of community resources available, as patients with cancer tend to require a multidisciplinary approach to management. Providers should anticipate, educate, manage, and provide frequent reassessment of sleep-wake disturbance that are often seen in patients with cancer. Early and appropriate interventions can provide improved outcomes in patients with cancer.

CLINICS CARE POINTS

- Sleep-wake disturbance is a common compliant in oncology settings and a multidimensional approach for management is useful.
- Sleep-wake disturbances present often with a myriad of other symptoms including, but not limited to, depression and anxiety.
- Unrecognized and untreated sleep-wake disturbance can result in long-term consequences to health.
- Identifying underlying etiologies is an important need for managing sleep-wake disturbances in oncology settings.
- Adverse effects of anticancer treatments, including endocrine therapy, can result in acute and chronic sleep-wake disturbances.
- Assessment of sleep-wake disturbances should occur routinely in oncology settings.

DISCLOSURE

The authors have nothing to disclose.

REFERENCES

1. O'Donnell JF. Insomnia in cancer patients. Clin Cornerstone 2004;6:S6–8.
2. Siefert ML, Hong F, Valcarce B, et al. Patient and clinician communication of self-reported insomnia during ambulatory cancer care clinic visits. Cancer Nurs 2014; 37:E51–9.
3. Woodward SC. Cognitive-behavioral therapy for insomnia in patients with cancer. Clin J Oncol Nurs 2011;15(4):E42–52.
4. Graci G. Pathogenesis and management of cancer-related insomnia. J Support Oncol 2005;3(5):349–59.
5. Mercadante S, Adile C, Aielli F, et al. Personalized goal for insomnia and clinical response in advanced cancer patients. Support Care Cancer 2020;28(3): 1089–96.
6. PDQ® Supportive and Palliative Care Editorial Board. PDQ Sleep Disorders. Bethesda, MD: National Cancer Institute. Available at: https://www.cancer.gov/about-cancer/treatment/side-effects/sleep-disorders-hp-pdq. Accessed October 14, 2020.
7. Bhaskar S, Hemavathy D, Prasad S. Prevalence of chronic insomnia in adult patients and its correlation with medical comorbidities. J Fam Med Prim Care 2016; 5(4):780–4.
8. Palesh OG, Roscoe JA, Mustian KM, et al. Prevalence, demographics, and psychological associations of sleep disruption in patients with cancer: University of Rochester Cancer Center-Community Clinical Oncology Program. J Clin Oncol 2010;28(2):292–8.
9. Guimond A-J, Ivers Hans, Savard Josee. Clusters of psychological symptoms in breast cancer: is there a common psychological mechanism? Cancer Nurs 2020; 43:343–53.
10. Savard J, Morin CM, Savard J, et al. Insomnia in the context of cancer: a review of a neglected problem. J Clin Oncol 2001;19(3):895–908.
11. Stone CR, Haig TR, Fiest KM, et al. The association between sleep duration and cancer-specific mortality: a systematic review and meta-analysis. Cancer Causes Control 2019;30(5):501–25.
12. Matthews E, Carter P, Page M, et al. Sleep-wake disturbance: a systematic review of evidence-based interventions for management in patients with cancer. Clin J Oncol Nurs 2018;22(1):37–52.
13. Papadopoulos D, Papadoudis A, Kiagia M, et al. Nonpharmacologic interventions for improving sleep disturbances in patients with lung cancer: a systematic review and meta-analysis. J Pain Symptom Manag 2018;55(5):1364–81.e5.
14. Hernandez Silva E, Lawler S, Langbecker D. The effectiveness of mHealth for self-management in improving pain, psychological distress, fatigue, and sleep in cancer survivors: a systematic review. J Cancer Surviv 2019;13(1):97–107.
15. Huang J, Han Y, Wei J, et al. The effectiveness of the Internet-based self-management program for cancer-related fatigue patients: a systematic review and meta-analysis. Clin Rehabil 2020;34(3):287–98.
16. Tang MF, Chiu HY, Xu X, et al. Walking is more effective than yoga at reducing sleep disturbance in cancer patients: A systematic review and meta-analysis of randomized controlled trials. Sleep Med Rev 2019;47:1–8.
17. Morin CM, Belleville G, Bélanger L, et al. The insomnia severity index: psychometric indicators to detect insomnia cases and evaluate treatment response. Sleep 2011;34(5):601–8.

18. Buysse DJ, Reynolds CF III, Monk TH, et al. The Pittsburgh Sleep Quality Index: a new instrument for psychiatric practice and research. Psychiatry Res 1989;28(2): 193–213.

19. Johns MW. A new method for measuring daytime sleepiness: the Epworth Sleepiness Scale. Sleep 1991;14(6):540–5.

20. Rizzo JD, Somerfield MR, Hagerty KL, et al. Use of epoetin and darbepoetin in patients with cancer: 2007 American Society of Clinical Oncology/American Society of Hematology clinical practice guideline update. J Clin Oncol 2008;26(1): 132–49.

21. The SHARE Approach. Content last reviewed October 2020. Agency for Healthcare Research and Quality, Rockville, MD. Available at: https://www.ahrq. gov/health-literacy/professional-training/shared-decision/index.html. Accessed December 15, 2020.

22. Schnipper LE, Bastian A. New frameworks to assess value of cancer care: strengths and limitations. Oncologist 2016;21(6):654–8.

23. Espie CA, Fleming L, Cassidy J, et al. Randomized controlled clinical effectiveness trial of cognitive behavior therapy compared with treatment as usual for persistent insomnia in patients with cancer. J Clin Oncol 2008;26(28):4651–8.

24. Dy SM, Apostol CC. Evidence-based approaches to other symptoms in advanced cancer. Cancer J 2010;16(5):507–13.

25. Page MS, Berger AM, Johnson LB. Putting evidence into practice: evidence-based interventions for sleep-wake disturbances. Clin J Oncol Nurs 2006; 10(6):753–83.

26. Centers for Disease Control and Prevention.

27. Sateia MJ, Buysse DJ, Krystal AD, et al. Clinical practice guideline for the pharmacologic treatment of chronic insomnia in adults: an American Academy of Sleep Medicine Clinical practice guideline. J Clin Sleep Med 2017;13(2):307–49.

28. Zhou L, Yu Y, Sun S, et al. Cry 1 regulates the clock gene network and promotes proliferation and migration via the Akt/P53/P21 pathway in human osteosarcoma cells. J Cancer 2018;9(14):2480–91.

29. Li Y, Cai S, Ling Y, et al. Association between total sleep time and all cancer mortality: non-linear dose-response meta-analysis of cohort studies. Sleep Med 2019; 60:211–8.

30. Charalambous A, Berger AM, Matthews E, et al. Cancer-related fatigue and sleep deficiency in cancer care continuum: concepts, assessment, clusters, and management. Support Care Cancer 2019;27(7):2747–53.

31. Kim H, Lee YW, Ju HJ, et al. An exploratory study on the effects of forest therapy on sleep quality in patients with gastrointestinal tract cancers. Int J Environ Res Public Health 2019;16(14):2449.

32. Harorani M, Davodabady F, Farahani Z, et al. The effect of Benson's relaxation response on sleep quality and anorexia in cancer patients undergoing chemotherapy: a randomized controlled trial. Complement therapies Med 2020;50: 102344.

33. Kurdi MS, Muthukalai SP. The efficacy of oral melatonin in improving sleep in cancer patients with insomnia: a randomized double-blind placebo-controlled study. Indian J Palliat Care 2016;22(3):295–300.

34. Heydarirad G, Keyhanmehr AS, Mofid B, et al. Efficacy of aromatherapy with Rosa damascena in the improvement of sleep quality of cancer patients: a randomized controlled clinical trial. Complement Therapies Clin Pract 2019;35: 57–61.

35. Wu LM, Amidi A, Valdimarsdottir H, et al. The effect of systematic light exposure on sleep in a mixed group of fatigued cancer survivors. J Clin Sleep Med 2018; 14(1):31–9.
36. Vinayak S, Dehkhoda F, Vinayak R. The effect of music therapy on sleep quality of cancer patients undergoing chemotherapy or radiotherapy: a randomized control trial. J Social Sci (Coes&rj-jss) 2017;6(4):734–43.
37. Liu XL, Cheng HL, Moss S, et al. Somatic acupoint stimulation for cancer-related sleep disturbance: a systematic review of randomized controlled trials. Evidence-based complementary and alternative medicine. eCAM 2020;2020:2591320.

Nature-Based Therapies for Sleep Disorders in People Living with Human Immunodeficiency Virus

Gibran Mancus, PhD, RN[a],*, Samantha V. Hill, MD, MPH[b],
Patricia Carter, PhD, RN, CNS[c], Pamela Payne-Foster, MD, MPH[d],
Mangala Krishnamurthy, MLIS, AHIP[e], Abigail Kazembe, PhD, RN[f],
Shameka L. Cody, PhD, AGNP-C[c]

KEYWORDS

- HIV • Nature therapy • Global health • Sleep disorders

KEY POINTS

- Poor sleep quality and insufficient quantity has been found to induce negative changes in immune system function.
- The impact sleep has on immune function and overall quality of life is best exemplified among people living with human immunodeficiency virus.
- Health care providers can provide information about the benefits of spending time in natural spaces as part of complementary therapy for sleep disorders.

PSYCHONEUROIMMUNOLOGY AND SLEEP DISORDERS
How Does Sleep Impact Life and Immune Function?

The relationships between sleep and immune function have been a focus of scientists and clinicians alike since the time of Aristotle in 350 BC.[1] Many advances in this relational understanding have occurred since then; however, much is still to learn. A preponderance of evidence supports the bidirectionality of sleep and the immune system. Immune system substances (eg, cytokines interleukin and tumor necrosis factor and

[a] Capstone College of Nursing, The University of Alabama, Box 870358, Tuscaloosa, AL 35487, USA; [b] Department of Pediatrics, Division of Adolescent Medicine, University of Alabama at Birmingham, Park Place 310, Birmingham, AL 35233, USA; [c] Capstone College of Nursing, The University of Alabama, Box 870358, Tuscaloosa, AL 30487, USA; [d] College of Community Health Sciences, The University of Alabama, Box 870358, Tuscaloosa, AL 30487, USA; [e] Rodgers Science and Engineering Library, The University of Alabama Libraries, Box 870266, Tuscaloosa, AL 35487, USA; [f] Neonatal and Reproductive Health Services, Kamuzu College of Nursing, The University of Malawi, Private Bag 1, Lilongwe, Malawi
* Corresponding author.
E-mail address: gmancus@ua.edu
Twitter: @GibranMancus (G.M.); @carter3236 (P.C.); @mkmurthyrarj (M.K.)

Nurs Clin N Am 56 (2021) 189–202
https://doi.org/10.1016/j.cnur.2021.02.002
0029-6465/21/© 2021 Elsevier Inc. All rights reserved.
nursing.theclinics.com

prostaglandins [PGs]) have been found to be key players in the regulation of sleep in animals and contribute to the regulation of non–rapid eye movement sleep amount and intensity in animals when infectious agents challenge the host defense.[2] It is hypothesized that these same cytokines and PGs also may be involved in sleep regulation and infection-induced human sleep responses. In chronic inflammatory or infectious states, it is important to consider how disease stage, symptom severity, and comorbid disorders may contribute to sleep changes observed.[3] Although work in humans is still in the early stages, the work of Karatas and colleagues[4] may illustrate the connection between immune system and chronic disease–associated sleep changes. This work shows that blunting the activity of specific inflammatory cytokines results in improved sleep.[4]

Experimental animal and human studies have demonstrated that manipulation of sleep quantity and quality affects a wide variety of immune system processes (eg, antibody levels, complement activation, leukocyte migration and distribution).[3] Consequently, it is understandable that sleep quality and quantity will affect the outcome of infections. This has been demonstrated through vaccination response in an experimental model of infection. Using this model, Kuo and Williams[5] demonstrated that quality sleep improved animal survival rates following infection and several human studies support that sleep deprivation increased the susceptibility to infections and reduced vaccination response.[6,7] Although the specific mechanisms underlying the effect of sleep on immune system performance are not well understood, the current literature supports the hypothesis that Slow Wave Sleep (SWS) may play a key role. Lange and colleagues[8] proposed that SWS induces an immune-supportive hormonal constellation that fosters and coordinates the migration of T cells and antigen-presenting cells to lymphatic tissues and supports communication between these cells, thus improving the adaptive immune response and stabilizing immunologic memory. The relationships between innate immune response and sleep quality are not well understood. Experimental studies support the exploration of mechanistic relationships; however, naturalistic studies, although less controlled, can inform interventions in the real world.

Studies conducted in the naturalistic setting reveal that total sleep duration above or below the recommended amount, as well as common sleep disturbances (eg, sleep apnea and insomnia) contribute to changes in inflammatory markers, immune cell counts, and cellular aging markers (eg, telomere length).[9] It is reasonable to consider that these types of immune system changes may be the link between sleep and disease risk; however, there is considerable variability between studies limiting the ability to compare findings.

Clinical Implications

Poor sleep quality and insufficient quantity has been found to induce negative changes in immune system function. Similarly, immune system changes, such as those seen in response to acute or chronic infections, result in changes to sleep regulation. It is a reasonable course of action for health care providers to target sleep as an integral part of disease prevention and treatment strategies. The following are some key points for health care providers to consider when working with patients diagnosed with chronic immune deficiency conditions (eg, human immunodeficiency virus [HIV]/AIDS).

- Sleep is a basic biological need of all species for optimal immune function.
- Sleep duration and quality contribute to susceptibility to illness and the ability to survive/recover from disease.

- To achieve optimal response to vaccinations, patients need adequate sleep before and after being vaccinated.
- Chronic sleep debt disrupts immune homeostasis and thus increases the risk for amplification of several diseases with immune dysregulation, such as HIV/AIDS.

Assessment

The first step in treatment for sleep disorders is to determine if they are present in the patient population. Given that sleep disturbances are common in the general population and nearly 70% of individuals with chronic medical conditions report problems with their sleep,[10] it is reasonable to presume that most individuals who health professionals encounter should be screened for sleep problems.

Deciding to screen is an easy choice, but knowing what instruments to use may not be (**Table 1**). As with most clinical activities, there are "gold standard" approaches and then there are realistic, practical, and accessible approaches. Table 1 provides a brief description of the common sleep disorders, the gold standard assessment, and the practical first-step approach.

Table 1
Sleep assessment tools

Disorder (Sleep Problem)	Gold Standard Assessment	Practical First-Step Approach
Sleep-disordered breathing: • Obstructive sleep apnea • Central sleep apnea	Polysomnography (PSG)-based sleep study administered in a sleep laboratory and scored by a sleep medicine specialist	Administer the STOP-BANG. This instrument assesses risk for sleep apnea through self-report (eg, observed gasping for air when sleeping) and physical characteristics (eg, neck size, hypertension). The score will determine if a sleep study is warranted.[11]
Insomnia • Difficulty falling asleep • Difficulty maintaining sleep (staying asleep) • Waking too early • Feeling unrefreshed when waking	Actigraphy combined with self-report sleep quality instruments (eg, Pittsburgh Sleep Quality Index [PSQI], Insomnia Severity Index [ISI])	The ISI is a 7-item empirically supported screen for insomnia that results in risk score.[12]
Excessive daytime sleepiness (EDS) • Complaints of ability to have enough energy to accomplish daily activities	Multiple-Sleep Latency Test administered in a sleep center[13]	Epworth Sleepiness Scale assesses the likelihood to fall asleep in 8 common situations. Score ranges from normal to severe.[14]
Sleep Movement Disorders • Restless limb syndrome (RLS) • Periodic limb movement (PLM)	PSG (sleep study) administered in a sleep laboratory to allow for video capture of sleep movements	RLS: self-report of noxious sensations in legs/arms when attempting to fall asleep. Relieved with movement/walking. PLM: Bed partner reports of repetitive movements (kicking/punching) during deep sleep

In addition to assessment of specific sleep disorders/complaints, a general sleep assessment can be made with a sleep diary. The Consensus Sleep Diary (CSD)[15] was developed through a collaboration of top sleep scientists to allow for standardization of prospective self-sleep monitoring. Incorporation of this type of ongoing self-sleep monitoring allows the individual to obtain a sense of their sleep-wake schedule and the factors that influence (positive and negative) sleep quality. This information can be reviewed during clinic visits to target and customize sleep focused interventions.

Conventional Sleep Disruption Treatments

As with assessment of sleep, the therapies or treatments are targeted to the underlying condition. However, given the complexities of chronic illnesses like HIV/AIDS, it is important to consider that individuals may present with comorbid sleep disorders (eg, obstructive sleep apnea and insomnia), that likely would require combination therapies. For the purposes of this presentation, Table 2 presents the therapies that are empirically supported for the most common conditions (sleep-disordered breathing and insomnia) listed previously.

Treatments for excessive daytime sleepiness and sleep movement disorders are primarily dependent on the underlying condition responsible for these symptoms. And although it is beyond the scope and purpose of this article to fully present this information, it is important for health care providers to assess for excessive daytime sleepiness and movement disorders to promote healthy sleep in their patients.

NATURE-BASED THERAPY

The physical environment is increasingly being recognized as a factor contributing to health and well-being. More specifically, the natural environment, parks, green spaces, and urban forests, have been suggested as supportive of health.[16] There are direct and indirect pathways that have been suggested.[17]

Table 2
Conventional sleep disruptions

Disorder (Sleep Problem)	High-Level Evidence	Moderate-Level Evidence
Sleep-disordered breathing: • Obstructive sleep apnea • Central sleep apnea	Continuous positive airway pressure. Delivers positive airway pressure to maintain airway patency.	• Dental appliances: support tongue and jaw position to maintain airway patency • Surgical intervention: removes excessive tissues to allow for airway patency • Positional aids: promotes side sleeping
Insomnia • Difficulty falling asleep • Difficulty maintaining sleep (staying asleep) • Waking too early • Feeling unrefreshed when waking	Cognitive behavioral therapy for insomnia (CBTI)[a] delivered by trained sleep specialist (one-on-one).	• Virtual CBTI: therapeutic elements delivered online

[a] Limited availability outside of metropolitan areas and may not be covered by healthcare insurance.

One pathway posits mental restoration from exposure to natural spaces. Stress from the social and built environment is thought to contribute to mental fatigue and nature is thought to mitigate stressful stimuli through passive engagement.[18] Nature engages the senses in a passive, nonthreatening way. When the wind blows through the branches of a trees, it makes a sound, people see the movement, smell the phytoncides, and feel the breeze on their faces. One or more combinations of these physical stimuli grab a person's attention in a way that is suggested to support parasympathetic activity, a more relaxed state, important for sleep. Another pathway involves how trees and vegetation in communities have been found to mitigate noise pollution. Noise pollution has been associated with increased stress response and disturbed sleep.[19,20] The mitigation of mental fatigue and noise pollution individually or collectively can decrease stress and potentially improve sleep. An alternative explanation may be the phytoncides of trees, specifically 3-Carene of the pine tree, which has been found to have anxiolytic effects.[21]

Persons living with higher levels of greenness, a measure of the green from the chlorophyll of plants, are less likely to have infants with low birth weights, liver cancer, kidney disease, and cardiovascular disease.[16,22,23] Findings among low-income communities show a positive relationship of greenness with the cortisol awakening response, an indicator of the hypothalamus-pituitary-adrenal axis response to physiologic stress.[24] Persons living with higher levels of greenness are less likely to have dehydroepiandrosterone (DHEA) in the bottom tenth percentile.[25] In one study among African American women at high risk of HIV, a positive association between the ratio of cortisol to DHEA, a potential biomarker of physiologic resilience, was found.[26]

In addition to associations with mental and physical health, healthy sleep has been found to have positive correlations with living with higher levels of green space and by intentionally spending time in forests and natural spaces.[27–29] In Japan. Shinrin-yoku or Forest Bathing, is the intentional act of spending time surrounded by forests or natural spaces. In a convenience sample of people in Japan, Morita and colleagues[27] found in a quasi-experimental study (n = 71) that 2 hours of forest walking significantly increased sleep time, sleep latency, and immobile time. In a cross-sectional study (n = 259,319) when compared with those living with 20% greenspace, those living with 80% or more green space had a 42% reduced risk of getting less than 6 hours of sleep rather than 8 hours.[28] In a nationally representative sample in the United States (n = 255,171), among those getting 21 to 29 days of insufficient sleep per month there was a 16% reduction in odds of exposure to natural amenities than those with 1 to 6 days.[29]

HUMAN IMMUNODEFICIENCY VIRUS IN RURAL POPULATIONS, FROM LOCAL TO GLOBAL, SOUTHEASTERN UNITED STATES TO SOUTHEASTERN MALAWI (STIGMA, VIOLENCE, LACK OF RESOURCES)

Clinical Applications: Sleep's Impact on Human Immunodeficiency Virus Health Outcomes

The importance of sleep quality and quantity is extremely important in the health outcomes among people living with HIV (PLWH). The following is a comparison of how sleep can impact the management of PLWH in 2 locations: the southern United States and southeastern Malawi. Since the HIV pandemic hit in the early 1980s, the epidemiology of the United States and the African continent has differed dramatically. Early in the US epidemic, HIV affected mainly white men, and in Africa, both African men and women were affected. Although the demographics over the decades have essentially remained the same in Africa, the demographics of HIV in the United States has shifted from white men to African American men and women. In addition, geographic shifts over the decades have shifted from urban centers along the coasts to the 16 states and District of Columbia that make up the South.[30] Fifty-one percent of new HIV cases annually in the United States (n = 37,968) are in the southern states and accounted for 47% of the US deaths (n = 15,807).[31,32] Southern states lag behind in providing quality HIV prevention services and care.[33,34]

Human immunodeficiency virus, from local to global, southeastern United States to southeastern Malawi (stigma, violence, lack of resources)

The heavy burden of HIV in the South, especially in those states considered the "Deep South," such as Alabama, Florida, Georgia, Louisiana, Mississippi, North Carolina, South Carolina, Tennessee, and Texas, is driven in part by socioeconomic factors like poverty and unemployment.[31] The South has the highest poverty rate and lowest median household income compared with other regions of the United States.[31] Both factors are associated with poorer health outcomes and may contribute to a higher concentration of HIV and other chronic diseases, like diabetes, in the region.

Additional reasons for the disproportionate burden in this region include lack of access to health services. Nearly half of all Americans without health insurance live in the South.[35] Medicaid is the largest source of coverage for people with HIV in the United States, but 9 of 16 states in the South have not expanded Medicaid.[36,37] In rural areas, people with or at risk for HIV face challenges in accessing consistent HIV prevention and treatment services, like lack of public transportation, longer travel time to receive care, and reduced availability of medical and social services compared with nonrural areas.[33] These places may also experience health care provider shortages and have fewer providers with expertise in treating HIV, which causes longer distances traveled and longer hours associated with visits. Access also may be affected by laws and policies that discriminate against disclosing one's status and fuel the epidemic.[33,34]

Last, cultural factors may also play a key role in driving the southern HIV epidemic. HIV stigma is pervasive in the South and is often associated with stigma around sexual orientation, substance use disorder, poverty, and sex work, and may limit people's willingness to disclose their HIV status or seek testing, care, or prevention services.[33,38] Stigma has been associated with lower or delayed access to care due to perceived discrimination from health care providers.[39,40]

East and Southern Africa are home to almost half of the global population of PLWH.[41] Malawi, with an HIV prevalence of 8.9%, is one the highest in the world among adults between the ages of 15 and 49. There are 1.1 million PLWH in Malawi. In 2019, there were 33,000 new HIV infections and 13,000 AIDS-related deaths. Seventy-nine percent of adults and 74% of children living with HIV are on antiretroviral treatment. Prevalence of HIV among women (12.8%) in Malawi in 2016 was found to be higher than that of men (8.2%).[41] Gender-based violence may be a driving force of the HIV epidemic, especially among women.[42] Lifetime reported intimate partner violence (IPV) in Malawi is 38%.[43] Although IPV does not cause HIV, violence is associated with high risk-taking behavior, which can increase the risk of infection.[44] HIV-related stigma exists with cultural factors regarding masculinity, morality, gender, and power.[45,46] Women are often the first to know their status from HIV testing at prenatal clinics. Fearful of telling their partners, women may or may not be able to take their medicine and may continue getting reinfected from their partner.

Furthermore, women have additional risk factors for HIV related to food insecurity. Almost 2 million people in Malawi are food insecure as of October 2020.[47] Gender inequality in Malawi leaves young girls more vulnerable when they are forced to drop out of school, increasing rates of sexual coercion and transactional sex. Even girls who have the finances to attend school, may not have the resources and social support to stay in school, leaving them vulnerable to exploitation.

CASE STUDIES
Alabama

S.S. is a 22-year-old man living with HIV who is virally suppressed and presenting to his HIV clinic with a chief complaint of worsening fatigue. He reports he just completed his substance use program for severe polysubstance use disorder (opioid, cannabis, and tobacco). During his treatment program, he was diagnosed with hypertension, posttraumatic stress disorder, and mood disorder. He was started on amlodipine 5 mg daily, atenolol 25 mg daily, prazosin 2 mg daily, suboxone 8 mg daily, quetiapine 300 mg daily, venlafaxine 150 mg daily, disulfiram 250 mg every night, and hydroxyzine 50 mg as needed in addition to continuing on Genvoya for HIV management. Since detoxing from opioids and cannabis, he has had difficulties sleeping, specifically difficulty falling and staying asleep during the 10-hour period he allots for rest at night. He reports a history of chronic fatigue, including a time 1 year ago when he was informed he was vitamin D deficient and required replacement vitamin D therapy. Associated factors with fatigue during that time included difficulties falling and staying asleep, stress, and poor access to food and transportation services, resulting in him seeing his therapist once a month.

He was diagnosed with HIV 1 year ago and resides in Alabama. Since he has been engaged in care, he has had unstable housing and was recently in a substance use facility for 3 months, but before and after has been homeless, sleeping at friends' houses. He is unemployed, with his highest level of education being a high school diploma. He self describes as a gay man, single, never married. He lives in a "food desert," which has decreased access to nutritious foods, and also has almost no income as he relies on the HIV clinic to provide him with food and resources. All of these conditions cause him stress.

The most likely explanation for this patient's worsening fatigue includes increasing stress after being released from a substance use program and probable vitamin D deficiency in the setting of food insecurity, which was confirmed with laboratory results. Changes in mood were also included in the differential, as this patient has a history of depression; however, per patient report, his mood improved since adjustment of his medications during substance use treatment and has remained stable since. Furthermore, this patient has always been compliant with his antiretrovirals and has an undetectable viral load (<20), making exacerbation or progression of HIV disease unlikely. Thyroid disease is also unlikely, as the patient did not have any other signs or symptoms commonly suggestive of thyroid disease.

The patient met with the in-clinic psychologist for a brief check-in regarding mental health. He also met with the in-clinic social worker to get re-plugged in with resources for food and transportation to primary care and mental health (psychiatry and psychology) appointments. Vitamin D replacement therapy was prescribed: one 50,000 IU pill once a week for an 8-week course. The patient returned for his regularly scheduled 3-month follow-up. He had completed his course of vitamin D and reported that his level of fatigue was back to his original baseline. Viral load was less than 20 copies/mL and CD4 count was unchanged from the previous visit.

Malawi

K.B. is a 38-year-old woman and a single mother of 3. She presents to a rural health clinic for reduced physical strength and drowsiness. Her village is 7 km from the nearest health center. Her body mass index is 21. Her CD4 count was 500 cells/mm^3 and viral load is undetectable on Tenofovir-Lamivudine-Dolutegravir. She started antiretroviral therapy 5 years ago after initial positive testing. K.B. got tested after the father of her children died. K.B.'s partner was physically, economically, and emotionally abusive.

K.B. has participated in training on natural medicine that included information about plants that support health through increased nutrition, preventing opportunistic infections, and remediating the environment. She has implemented much of what she learned by cultivating plants around her home. She has created a kitchen garden just outside her house, which includes supplements to her diet, such as onions, tomatoes, cabbage, pumpkin, sweet potatoes, pigeon peas, and ground nuts. She has a few fruit trees, including tamarind, passion fruit, pineapple, mango, papaya, guava, baobab, avocado, lemon, and orange. She also has a medicinal garden with cayenne, garlic, ginger, lemon grass, hibiscus, neem, and aloe vera. The evidence for most of these herbs is limited.[48] Lemongrass tea has been found to reduce anxiety, promote sleep, and reduce inflammation. Garlic has been found to stimulate the immune system. Ginger has been found to stimulate appetite, alleviate nausea and vomiting, and reduce inflammation. Neem has been found to treat fungal infections on the skin and oral hygiene.[48]

K.B. also cultivates *Moringa oleifera* trees. She uses them as fencing to keep her neighbors' goats out of the garden. Furthermore, she dries and powders the leaves of the Moringa tree and uses it as a nutritional supplement[49] and sells the extra. She uses the seeds to treat her water from the village shallow well. The moringa trees also prevent erosion of her land when there are heavy rains.

K.B. volunteers as an expert client in a peer adherence support program, which provides her a small monetary stipend. Due to erratic rainfall this year, her maize (corn) production is of concern. The harvest season begins in the end of April. As part of a village savings and loan, she and some other women from the village savings and loan borrowed money to plant sweet potatoes to sell on the market.

Although K.B. has made huge changes in her life since the death of her husband, the trauma still impacts her today. K.B. does not have access to mental health services and limited social support. She has the community of expert clients for some social support but the pandemic has limited interactions. The garden that she has created around her house in addition to the support that it provides for her physical health also is something that she enjoys. K.B. does not sleep well, often waking up with nightmares. When she cannot sleep, she goes outside into her garden and drinks tea she makes from herbs in her garden. Her favorite tea is a mixture of lemongrass and hibiscus.

DISCUSSION

These cases are derived from the clinical and research expertise of the authors of this paper and represent both similarities and differences among PLWH. **Table 3** shows a comparison of HIV between Alabama and Malawi and factors that may play a role in sleep disorders. There are demographic and gender differences between PLWH in Malawi and Alabama. Issues such as IPV, homelessness, ruralness, and stigma (HIV-, sex-, sexuality-related) appear to have similarities across both populations and should be considered in addressing sleep disorders in HIV clients.

Although the Alabama case presented occurred from an urban area, one thing that makes the Deep South's HIV epidemic unique from the epidemic in the rest of the United States is that challenges to care in urban and rural areas are extremely similar, with the extent depending on rurality. For instance, the challenges related to provider access, as well as increased poverty and other social barriers, such as decreased

Table 3
Contrasting HIV and sleep impacts in Alabama versus Malawi

Topic:	HIV in Alabama	HIV in Malawi	Sleep Considerations
Viral suppression	• 62% of PLWH are virally suppressed	• 69% of PLWH are virally suppressed	• Poor sleep may be consequence of long-term use of antiretrovirals[50]
Gender-related differences	• Greater prevalence among young men having sex with men	• Greater prevalence among heterosexual young women (age 25–29)	• Women report more sleep disturbance than men.
IPV prevalence	• High prevalence of IPV	• High prevalence of IPV	• Data are limited, so IPV may be a key factor in sleep disturbance
Stigma	• Stigma with sexual orientation and fear of disclosure	• Homosexuality is criminalized. • Risk excommunication from church/family/friends	• Psychosocial factors
Sex workers	• Sex workers are often victims of abuse, homeless, and/or transient	• Sex workers are often victims of abuse • Sex work is legal in Malawi • Sex workers may be evicted and denied housing due to their occupation	• Psychosocial and environmental factors • Unstable sleeping environment • Exposed to extreme temperatures • Unsanitary conditions
Impact of clinic rurality	• Lack of access to specialized care for PLWH in rural areas • Farther distance to travel • Challenges with Internet connections for telehealth	• Rural clinics are unevenly distributed with low physician to population ratio	• Limited opportunity to discuss sleep issues with provider

Abbreviations: HIV, human immunodeficiency virus; IPV, intimate partner violence; PLWH, people living with HIV.

transportation and increased food insecurity, occur in both rural and urban areas in the Deep South, but may be even greater for individuals living in rural areas. Alabama is predominately rural, where 55 of 67 counties are rural.[51] In 2018, 84% of Malawians resided in rural areas.[52] Alabama also has an African American population of 25%, representing one of the states with the largest African American population.[30] This is important for this case, because sleep disorders, particularly, sleep apnea, may be disproportionately represented in the African American population due to disproportionate rates of other comorbidities.[53]

The spareness of clinicians reporting direct HIV-related sleep issues suggests this issue is not on the immediate radar of most clinicians who take care of PLWH in Alabama. Prevalence of sleep disorder among PLWH are more prevalent than in the general public.[54] This may be especially true for those who treat patients in rural areas, where there is a lack of specialty care (infectious disease specialists) and where patients with HIV must rely on more primary care or have to travel long distances to get comprehensive care. For example, screening tools, such as the Insomnia Severity Scale, which provides prompts for clinicians to question about sleep-related issues in patients with HIV are rarely used.[54] Furthermore, this questionnaire could miss more vague symptoms, which tend to be related to sleep, such as (1) chronic pain, (2) frequent awakenings, (3) falling asleep later, and (4) daytime sleepiness.

Both cases emphasized the impact of food insecurity, as both clients lived in "food deserts." The client in Malawi used her education in natural medicine and techniques to begin planting and farming as a way to supplement her nutritional requirements. The client in Alabama did not have access to the knowledge, skills, or space to grow his own food and had to rely on resources provided by his health care team to supplement his nutritional requirements. In addition, this client also received vitamin D supplementation. Interestingly, both clients also experienced stress related to their food insecurity, highlighting that the absences or lack of availability of foods may have both physical and emotional impacts on sleep. Nutritional deficiencies should be thoroughly explored in HIV clients and also should be considered as underlying issues in sleep disorders.

The other related symptoms that clinicians should pay attention to are psychiatric or psychosocial issues. The Alabama case highlighted psychological distress associated in general with sexual orientation and substance use. One study among PLWH in 3 southern US states where 65% of respondents were African American men and approximately half lived in rural areas revealed the mean psychological distress score on a standardized scale was higher than that of the general population.[33] It is reported that as many as 30% of HIV cases in the United States are associated with 1 or more substance use and abuse disorders.[55] In addition, it has been theorized that African American populations are often more religious, particularly those in the Deep South, and that reconciling religiosity and sexual orientation issues may contribute to sleep disorders.[56] In Malawi, sexual orientation represents both religious and legal issues. The Malawi case highlighted how past traumas, such as IPV, can continue to impact sleep even after the inciting event has been removed.

The integration of nature-based therapies in rural areas create many challenges and roles for health care providers. Even though there is the potential for those living in rural areas to have more access to green space, this is not always the case. In Malawi, rural areas have been heavily deforested due to the need for fuel for cooking and timber for building. In 2018, more than 38 million tons of forest products were removed from the land in Alabama. In both Malawi and Alabama, there are continual efforts to plant trees on the land; however, a significant portion of the tree planting is centered on the agroforestry industry. These trees are not there for the physical and mental health benefit of the people living nearby. These are not areas for forest bathing. Safety is also a challenge in both Malawi and Alabama with regard to opportunities to potentially enjoy nature. Being able to safely walk or sit in natural spaces that potentially can support health depends on a multitude of factors. Land ownership and right of way can limit access. Domesticated and wild animals, including dogs, can be a physical or psychological threat. Even when people have access, there may be a knowledge gap with regard to potential benefits. Health care providers can provide information about the benefits of spending time in natural spaces as part of complementary therapy for sleep disorders. In addition, health care providers can advocate with policy makers for the creation and protection of natural spaces, especially in communities that have limited access.

Last, because Coronavirus Disease 2019 (COVID-19) has affected the world globally, we should pay attention to its effects on patients with HIV, especially around issues of sleep disorders. COVID-19 had no impact on the status of the Alabama patient because he was already in a difficult financial, nutritional, mental health, and social support state before the pandemic. With regard to the Malawi case, COVID-19 has exacerbated access to medications and support because of increase stigma and fear. K.B. is concerned about her potential increased risk from COVID-19 and misinformation being spread that people with HIV are "Corona Carriers."

SUMMARY

The impact sleep has on immune function and overall quality of life is best exemplified among PLWH. Although the literature continues to show the impact sleep has on individuals' immune systems, recognition of how diagnoses with immunologic disorders such as HIV can impact sleep is just as important. Clinicians should be trained in screening and addressing factors that impact sleep, such as stigma, IPV, and regular stressors of living in today's society as a part of a comprehensive history and physical to provide specific treatment plans to identify and treat sleep disorders. Increasing awareness of sleep's impact on the health outcomes of PLWH is crucial in order to provide comprehensive, holistic treatment to the "whole" person.

CLINICS CARE POINTS

- Health care providers should integrate sleep disorder screenings into their practice.
- Providers can screen clients for their access and use of natural spaces.
- Recommend clients to engage with nature in their life for 10 to 50 minutes daily. Possible opportunities include trees, planters, potted plants, and parks. This can be done by either sitting or walking in those spaces.
- Recommend clients immerse themselves in natural spaces for 1 hour weekly. Possible locations include nearby parks, gardens, and trails.
- Providers can educate themselves on natural spaces in the catchment area. Create brochures that highlight places where clients can find places to be surrounded by nature.
- Recommend clients to spend 1 week a year immersed in nature as much as possible (no technology). Possible opportunities include camping and retreats (many have costs, but some have scholarships). Semi-immersion close to home can come from intentionally spending as much time during a week outside immersed in natural spaces in the community.
- Recommend clients to increase nature in their world. This can include having potted plants in their home, planters outside and planting trees. Many cities will provide trees free to community members who will help to water the plant until it gets established (2–3 years).
- Consider supporting greening interventions and policies in your community as an extension of your practice to promote health (ie, planting trees along streets).
- People with allergies will want to identify plants and trees that are more hypoallergenic.

DISCLOSURE

The authors have nothing to disclose.

REFERENCES

1. Aristotle. (350 BCE). On Sleep and Sleeplessness (J. I. Beare, Trans.). In. Cambridge (MA): Massachusetts Institute of Technology. Available at: http://classics.mit.edu//Aristotle/sleep.html.

2. Oishi Y, Yoshida K, Scammell TE, et al. The roles of prostaglandin E2 and D2 in lipopolysaccharide-mediated changes in sleep. Brain Behav Immun 2015;47: 172–7.

3. Besedovsky L, Lange T, Haack M. The sleep-immune crosstalk in health and disease. Physiol Rev 2019;99(3):1325–80.

4. Karatas G, Bal A, Yuceege M, et al. The evaluation of sleep quality and response to anti-tumor necrosis factor α therapy in rheumatoid arthritis patients. Clin Rheumatol 2017;36(1):45–50.

5. Kuo TH, Williams JA. Increased sleep promotes survival during a bacterial infection in Drosophila. Sleep 2014;37(6):1077–1086D. https://doi.org/10.5665/sleep.3764.

6. Lambert ND, Ovsyannikova IG, Pankratz VS, et al. Understanding the immune response to seasonal influenza vaccination in older adults: a systems biology approach. Expert Rev Vaccin 2012;11(8):985–94.

7. Lange T, Dimitrov S, Bollinger T, et al. Sleep after vaccination boosts immunological memory. J Immunol 2011;187(1):283.

8. Lange T, Dimitrov S, Fehm H, et al. Shift of monocyte function toward cellular immunity during sleep. Arch Intern Med 2006;166(16):1695–700. https://doi.org/10.1001/archinte.166.16.1695.

9. Foster SB, Lu M, Glaze DG, et al. Associations of cytokines, sleep patterns, and neurocognitive function in youth with HIV infection. Clin Immunol 2012;144(1): 13–23.

10. Ancoli-Israel S. The impact and prevalence of chronic insomnia and other sleep disturbances associated with chronic illness. Am J Manag Care 2006;12(8 Suppl):S221–9.

11. Chung F, Abdullah HR, Liao P. STOP-bang questionnaire: a practical approach to screen for obstructive sleep apnea. Chest 2016;149(3):631–8.

12. Morin CM, Belleville G, Bélanger L, et al. The insomnia severity index: psychometric indicators to detect insomnia cases and evaluate treatment response. Sleep 2011;34(5):601–8.

13. Littner MR, Kushida C, Wise M, et al. Practice parameters for clinical use of the multiple sleep latency test and the maintenance of wakefulness test. Sleep 2005;28(1):113–21.

14. Pilcher JJ, Switzer FS 3rd, Munc A, et al. Psychometric properties of the Epworth Sleepiness Scale: a factor analysis and item-response theory approach. Chronobiol Int 2018;35(4):533–45.

15. Carney CE, Buysse DJ, Ancoli-Israel S, et al. The consensus sleep diary: standardizing prospective sleep self-monitoring. Sleep 2012;35(2):287–302.

16. James P, Hart JE, Banay RF, et al. Exposure to greenness and mortality in a nationwide prospective cohort study of women. Environ Health Perspect 2016; 124(9):1344–52.

17. Kuo M. How might contact with nature promote human health? Promising mechanisms and a possible central pathway. Front Psychol 2015;6(1093).

18. Berman MG, Jonides J, Kaplan S. The cognitive benefits of interacting with nature. Psychol Sci 2008;19(12):1207–12.

19. Halperin D. Environmental noise and sleep disturbances: a threat to health? Sleep Sci 2014;7(4):209–12.

20. Spreng M. Possible health effects of noise induced cortisol increase. Noise Health 2000;2(7):59–64.

21. Woo J, Yang H, Yoon M, et al. 3-carene, a phytoncide from pine tree has a sleep-enhancing effect by targeting the GABA(A)-benzodiazepine receptors. Exp Neurobiol 2019;28(5):593–601.

22. Hystad P, Davies HW, Frank L, et al. Residential greenness and birth outcomes: evaluating the influence of spatially correlated built-environment factors. Environ Health Perspect 2014;122(10):1095–102.

23. Li Q, Otsuka T, Kobayashi M, et al. Acute effects of walking in forest environments on cardiovascular and metabolic parameters. Eur J Appl Physiol 2011;111:2845–53.

24. Roe JJ, Thompson CW, Aspinall PA, et al. Green space and stress: evidence from cortisol measures in deprived urban communities. Int J Environ Res Public Health 2013;10(9):4086–103.

25. Egorov AI, Griffin SM, Converse RR, et al. Vegetated land cover near residence is associated with reduced allostatic load and improved biomarkers of neuroendocrine, metabolic and immune functions. Environ Res 2017;158:508–21.

26. Mancus G, Cimino AN, Hasan MZ, et al. Residential Greenness Positively Associated with the Cortisol to DHEA Ratio among Urban-Dwelling African American Women at Risk for HIV. J Urban Health 2020. https://doi.org/10.1007/s11524-020-00492-0.

27. Morita E, Imai M, Okawa M, et al. A before and after comparison of the effects of forest walking on the sleep of a community-based sample of people with sleep complaints. BioPsychoSocial Med 2011;5(1):13.

28. Astell-Burt T, Feng X, Kolt GS. Does access to neighbourhood green space promote a healthy duration of sleep? Novel findings from a cross-sectional study of 259 319 Australians. BMJ Open 2013;3(8):e003094.

29. Grigsby-Toussaint DS, Turi KN, Krupa M, et al. Sleep insufficiency and the natural environment: Results from the US Behavioral Risk Factor Surveillance System survey. Prev Med 2015;78:78–84.

30. USCENSUS. US census bureau quick Facts, Alabama, United States. Washington, DC: US Department of Commerce; 2019.

31. USCDC. HIV in the Southern United States. Atlanta (GA): US Centers for Disease Control; 2019.

32. Hiv.gov. U.S. statistics: fast facts 2020. Available at: https://www.hiv.gov/hiv-basics/overview/data-and-trends/statistics. Accessed March 23, 2021.

33. Reif S, Safley D, McAllaster C, et al. State of HIV in the US Deep South. J Community Health 2017;42(5):844–53.

34. Adimora AA, Ramirez C, Schoenbach VJ, et al. Policies and politics that promote HIV infection in the Southern United States. AIDS 2014;28(10).

35. Blumberg LJ, HJ, Karpman M, et al. Characteristics of the remaining uninsured: an update. Robert Wood Johnson Foundation and the Urban Institute. Princeton (NJ): Urban Institute; 2018.

36. The affordable care act and HIV/AIDS 2019. Available at: https://www.hiv.gov/federal-response/policies-issues/the-affordable-care-act-and-hiv-aids. Accessed March 23, 2021.

37. Kaiser Family Foundation. Status of state Medicaid expansion decisions: interactive map. San Francisco: Kaiser Family Foundation; 2019. Available at: https://www.kff.org/medicaid/issue-brief/status-of-state-medicaid-expansion-decisions-interactive-map/.

38. Foster PH. Use of Stigma, fear, and denial in development of a framework for prevention of HIV/AIDS in rural African American communities. Fam Community Health 2007;30(4):318–27.

39. Stringer KL, Turan B, McCormick L, et al. HIV-related stigma among healthcare providers in the Deep South. AIDS Behav 2016;20(1):115–25.

40. Batey DS, Whitfield S, Mulla M, et al. Adaptation and implementation of an intervention to reduce HIV-Related stigma among healthcare workers in the United States: piloting of the FRESH Workshop. AIDS Patient Care and STDs 2016; 30(11):519–27.

41. UNAIDS. UNAIDS Malawi country overview. Geneva (Switzerland): United Nations Program on HIV and AIDS; 2020.

42. Jewkes RK, Dunkle K, Nduna M, et al. Intimate partner violence, relationship power inequity, and incidence of HIV infection in young women in South Africa: a cohort study. The Lancet 2010;376(9734):41–8.

43. UNWomen. Global database on violence against women: Malawi. 2016. Available at: https://evaw-global-database.unwomen.org/en/countries/africa/malawi?%20formofviolence56e5dd05b2c3440798afe78c32f97d57f. Accessed March 23, 2021.

44. Durevall D, Lindskog A. Intimate partner violence and HIV in ten sub-Saharan African countries: what do the Demographic and Health Surveys tell us? Lancet Glob Health 2015;3(1):e34–43.

45. Lindgren T, Rankin SH, Rankin WW. Malawi women and HIV: socio-cultural factors and barriers to prevention. Womens Health 2005;41(1):69–86.

46. Hershow RB, Zimba CC, Mweemba O, et al. Perspectives on HIV partner notification, partner HIV self-testing and partner home-based HIV testing by pregnant and postpartum women in antenatal settings: a qualitative analysis in Malawi and Zambia. J Int AIDS Soc 2019;22(Suppl 3):e25293.

47. UNFAO. Country briefs Malawi. Rome (Italy): Food and Agriculture Organization of the United Nations; 2020.

48. Memorial Sloan Kettering Cancer Center. About herbs, botanicals & other products. 2020. Available at: https://www.mskcc.org/cancer-care/diagnosis-treatment/symptom-management/integrative-medicine/herbs. Accessed March 23, 2021.

49. Abdull Razis AF, Ibrahim MD, Kntayya SB. Health benefits of *Moringa oleifera*. Asian Pac J Cancer Prev 2014;15(20):8571–6.

50. Dalwadi DA, Ozuna L, Harvey BH, et al. Adverse neuropsychiatric events and recreational use of efavirenz and other HIV-1 antiretroviral drugs. Pharmacol Rev 2018;70(3):684–711.

51. Alabama Rural Health Association. Analysis of urban vs. rural. Troy (AL): Alabama Rural Health Association; 2020.

52. National Statistical office of Malawi. Malawi in figures. Zomba, Malawi: Government of Malawi; 2020.

53. Johnson DA, Guo N, Rueschman M, et al. Prevalence and correlates of obstructive sleep apnea among African Americans: the Jackson Heart Sleep Study. Sleep 2018;41(10):zsy154.

54. Gutierrez J, Tedaldi EM, Armon C, et al. Sleep disturbances in HIV-infected patients associated with depression and high risk of obstructive sleep apnea. SAGE Open Med 2019;7. 2050312119842268.

55. Jehan S, Zizi F, Pandi-Perumal SR, et al. Obstructive sleep apnea and obesity: implications for public health. Sleep Med Disord 2017;1(4):00019.

56. Pew Research Cener. A religious portrait of African-Americans. Washington, DC: Pew Research Center; 2009.

Sleep and Inflammation

Sleep and Metabolic Syndrome

Eileen R. Chasens, PhD, RN[a],*, Christopher C. Imes, PhD, RN[b],
Jacob K. Kariuki, PhD, AGNP-BC[a], Faith S. Luyster, PhD[a], Jonna L. Morris, PhD, RN[a],
Monica M. DiNardo, PhD, ANP-BC, CDCES[c], Cassandra M. Godzik, PhD, APRN[d],
Bomin Jeon, MSN, RN, PhD candidate[a], Kyeongra Yang, PhD, MPH, RN[e]

KEYWORDS

- Metabolic syndrome • Short sleep duration • Circadian misalignment • Insomnia
- Sleep apnea

KEY POINTS

- Metabolic syndrome and impaired sleep share many of the same phenotypical characteristics and risk factors, including increased prevalence in middle-aged and older adults, obesity with central adiposity, hypertension, dyslipidemia, and hyperglycemia.
- There is a U-shaped association between sleep duration and health outcomes: individuals with short ($\leq$5 h/d) or long ($\geq$9 h/d) sleep duration showed higher risk for metabolic syndrome than those with normal sleep duration (7–8 h/d).
- Misaligned sleep and nighttime eating have negative effects on cardiometabolic factors, such as adiposity, glucose, and cholesterol.
- Insomnia is found to be a risk factor for the development of metabolic syndrome. Specific insomnia symptoms, primarily difficulties in initiating and maintaining sleep, are associated with the metabolic syndrome and its components.
- Sleep disorders including obstructive sleep apnea are prevalent in persons with metabolic syndrome. A sleep assessment should be part of the health provider's routine assessment in persons with metabolic syndrome.

INTRODUCTION

Health, according to the World Health Organization, is conceptualized not as only the absence of disease but also as full human physical, emotional, mental, and social function.[1] Obtaining an adequate quantity of restorative sleep each night is a basic

---

[a] School of Nursing, University of Pittsburgh, 3500 Victoria Street, Suite 415, Pittsburgh, PA 15261, USA; [b] School of Nursing, University of Pittsburgh, 3500 Victoria Street, Suite 336, Pittsburgh, PA 15261, USA; [c] Center for Heath Equity, Research and Promotion, VA Pittsburgh Healthcare System, 151C University Drive, Pittsburgh, PA 15201, USA; [d] Department of Psychiatry, Dartmouth College and Dartmouth-Hitchcock Medical Center, 46 Centerra Parkway, Lebanon, NH 03766, USA; [e] School of Nursing, Rutgers, The State University of New Jersey, 65 Bergen Street, Room 1025E, Newark, NJ 07107, USA
* Corresponding author.
E-mail address: chasense@pitt.edu

Nurs Clin N Am 56 (2021) 203–217
https://doi.org/10.1016/j.cnur.2020.10.012
0029-6465/21/© 2020 Elsevier Inc. All rights reserved.

nursing.theclinics.com

requisite for human health; however, the function of sleep in maintaining metabolic homeostasis has not been elucidated fully. During the past 20 years, there has been an increased study of the role of inadequate sleep and sleep disorders on cardiometabolic factors, such as the pathogenesis of obesity, hypertension, dyslipidemia, and hyperglycemia. This review examines studies on impaired sleep (ie, insufficient, fragmented, or poor quality), sleep disorders (ie, obstructive sleep apnea [OSA] and insomnia), and circadian misalignment of sleep (eg, evening chronotype, social jet lag, or shift work) and metabolic syndrome (MetS).

Many factors may be associated with the epidemic increase in prevalence of sleep disorders in the United States, including the aging population and modern lifestyle factors that do not favor sleep and contribute to overweight and obesity. Sleep-disordered breathing (SDB) and nocturnal breathing disorders that include OSA, central sleep apnea, and nocturnal hypoventilation syndrome also are prevalent. Depending on age and disease severity, the estimated prevalence of mild SDB ranges from 24.0% to 83.8% in men and from 9.0% to 76.6% in women. Moderate to severe SDB ranges from 7.2% to 67.2% in men compared with 4.0% to 50.9% in women, in whom the rate of SDB increases by up to 6% after menopause, approaching the rate for men.[2] Likewise, 20% to 40% of United States adults report insomnia symptoms, that is, having difficulty initiating sleep, maintaining sleep, early morning wakening, or nonrefreshing sleep, and 9% to 15% have insomnia symptoms accompanied by daytime sleepiness or fatigue.[3,4]

Over the past 20 years, the prevalence of MetS in United States adults has increased in parallel with that of obesity. The prevalence of MetS increased from 25.3% to 36.9% between 1988 and 2016.[5,6] A comparative study of National Health and Nutrition Examination Survey (NHANES) data during that time period found that the prevalence of obesity (body mass index [BMI] $\geq$30 kg/m^2) in men increased from 27.5% to 43.0% and the rate of severe obesity (BMI $\geq$40 kg/m^2) more than doubled, from 3.1% to 6.8%. Rates of obesity among adult women increased from 33.4% to 41.9% and from 6.2% to 11.5% for severe obesity.[7]

The article describes (1) epidemiologic evidence on the prevalence and association of impaired sleep with MetS, (2) potential mechanisms where impaired sleep desynchronizes and worsens metabolic control, and (3) interventions to improve sleep and potentially improve MetS. Although there are a vast number of studies that separately examine each different condition that contribute to MetS, only studies in adults that consider MetS as the whole cluster of conditions are discussed.

METABOLIC SYNDROME: DEFINITION AND PREVALENCE

MetS is a cluster of endogenous risk factors for development of cardiometabolic disease: increased triglycerides (TGs), decreased high-density lipoprotein cholesterol (HDL), increased blood pressure (BP), increased central adiposity, and increased fasting glucose.[8,9] Although each cardiometabolic risk factor is known to independently increase the likelihood of developing diabetes and/or cardiovascular disease (CVD), the co-occurrence of these interrelated risk factors is known to compound the risk.[10,11] Various organizations have supported slightly different definitions of MetS. The following 3 definitions commonly are used for clinical and research purposes: National Cholesterol Education Program Adult Treatment Panel III (ATP III), International Diabetes Federation (IDF), and American Heart Association (AHA) and National Heart, Lung, and Blood Institute (NHLBI) (**Table 1**).

Due to the heterogeneity inherent in the diagnostic criteria employed by various expert panels, the true global and country specific prevalence of MetS remains uncertain, and current estimates vary based on the criterion used.[12] Despite these limitations, multiple studies have estimated the incidence and prevalence of MetS. It is estimated that approximately 25% of the world population has MetS.[12] In the United States, estimates using the 2003 to 2006 NHANES data suggest that the overall age-adjusted prevalence of MetS is approximately 34% based on the ATP III criteria.[13] In this study, non-Hispanic white men had a higher prevalence of MetS (37%) compared with non-Hispanic black men (25%), but there were no significant differences in prevalence among women based on race/ethnicity.[13] The prevalence of MetS (IDF criteria) in the United States has increased from 1988 to 2012, regardless of sociodemographic characteristics (such as ethnicity, gender, and age) and the prevalence of MetS was 34.2% during the period 2007 to 2012.[6] In 2015 to 2016, the prevalence (ATP III criteria) increased to 36.9% among adults aged 20 years or older and to 50.4% among those aged at least 60 years.[5]

The interplay of this cluster of metabolic aberrancies, spurred on by an accumulation of visceral fat and linked to insulin resistance, increases the risk of type 2 diabetes (T2DM), atherosclerosis, and all-cause mortality.[14] Each component of MetS is an independent risk factor for cardiometabolic disease, a group of highly prevalent, interrelated conditions that includes cardiovascular disease (CVD) including coronary heart disease, stroke, and hypertension, and metabolic conditions such as obesity, T2DM, and non-alcoholic fatty liver disease (NAFLD). The combination of these factors elevates rates and severity of systemic inflammation and cardiovascular conditions. Having MetS is associated with a 5-fold increase in the risk of T2DM and a 2-fold risk of developing CVD over a period of 5 to 10 years.[15]

SLEEP DURATION AND METABOLIC SYNDROME

Adequate sleep duration, the amount of time spent sleeping within a 24-hour period of time to maintain optimal health and well-being, ranges from 7 hours to 9 hours for adults and 7 hours to 8 hours for older adults.[16] A review of studies with population-level data found the prevalence of objectively measured short sleep duration, that is, less than 6 hours, ranged from 22.1% to 53.3% of United States adults[17] whereas 9.2% of the population report having long sleep duration ($\geq$9 hours).[18] Reasons for short sleep duration include long work hours; early morning awakening because of long commutes to work, house and childcare responsibilities in working parents; and increased use of technology in the evening with sleep delayed.[19] A study using NHANES 2007 to 2008 data examined the association of sleep duration, ranging from very short (<5 h/night) to long ($\geq$9 h/night), by social determinant factors, with normal sleep duration (7 h/night to 8 h/night) as the reference.[20] Shorter sleep durations were significantly more likely in persons who were African American, Hispanics/Latino, Asians, low income, low education level, with public insurance, or with low food security (P<.05).[20]

Multiple studies report a U-shaped distribution between persons with normal sleep duration and those with short or long sleep duration and worse health outcomes (ie, obesity, T2DM, and hypertension).[21,22] A meta-analysis evaluated prospective studies (N = 15) that had baseline data on sleep duration and data from at least a 3-year follow-up period. This study found a significantly increased risk for short duration for incidence and death from CVD and stroke; long sleep duration had significantly increased risk for incidence and death for cardiac heart disease, stroke, and total CVD.[21] Although long sleep duration is associated with increased morbidity, it is hypothesized that the association between long sleep and poor cardiovascular

Table 1
Definitions of metabolic syndrome

	National Cholesterol Education Program Adult Treatment Panel III, 2001	International Diabetes Federation, 2006	The American Heart Association and the National Heart, Lung, and Blood Institute, 2005
Mandatory risk factor	None	Central obesity (waist circumference with ethnicity specific value: $\geq$102 cm for men; $\geq$88 cm for women in whites and $\geq$90 cm for men, $\geq$80 cm for female in Asians) OR BMI >30 kg/m^2	None
Additional risk factors	At least 3 of the following risk factors: Central adiposity (waist circumference >102 cm for men; >88 cm for women)	Any 2 of the following risk factors:	At least 3 of the following risk factors: Central adiposity (waist circumference >102 cm for men; >88 cm for women)
	Elevated fasting TGs ($\geq$150 mg/dL)	Elevated TGs ($\geq$150 mg/dL) OR Drug treatment	Elevated TGs ($\geq$150 mg/dL) OR Drug treatment
	Low fasting HDL cholesterol <40 mg/dL for men or <50 mg/dL for women)	Low HDL cholesterol (<40 mg/dL for men or <50 mg/dL for women) OR Drug treatment	Low HDL cholesterol (<40 mg/dL for men or <50 mg/dL for women) OR Drug treatment
	High BP ($\geq$130/85 mm Hg)	High BP ($\geq$130/85 mm Hg) OR Drug treatment	High BP ($\geq$130/85 mm Hg) OR Drug treatment
	Elevated fasting blood glucose levels (>110 mg/dL)	Elevated fasting blood glucose levels ($\geq$100 mg/dL) OR Previously diagnosed T2DM	Elevated fasting blood glucose levels ($\geq$100 mg/dL) OR Drug treatment

outcomes is an indicator of poor health rather than a risk factor or potential mechanism for negative health outcomes.[18,21]

A study with the 2013 to 2014 NHANES data of a population-level sample examined the association between sleep duration and MetS severity (ATP III criteria).[22] In this study, individuals sleeping 7 hours to 7.5 hours per night showed the lowest risk for MetS. In a U-shaped association between sleep duration and MetS, those sleeping less than 7 hours or more than 7 hours were at higher risk than those sleeping 7 hours, and those sleeping 5 hours or 9 hours showed similar risk.

CIRCADIAN MISALIGNMENT AND METABOLIC SYNDROME

Sleeping and eating outside of the normal light-dark cycle and out of phase with the central clock cause circadian misalignment.[23] Circadian misalignment is associated with impaired glucose control and increased inflammatory markers. Individuals with long-term circadian misalignment are at increased risk for an elevated BMI, diabetes, CVD, and stroke.[24]

Chronotype, social demands, and work schedules are factors that have an impact on the circadian system and contribute to circadian misalignment. Chronotype is the natural variation in circadian rhythms that manifests in preferred bedtime and peak performance.[25] There are 3 basic chronotypes: early (morning), intermediate, and late (evening). Numerous factors have an impact on chronotype and it changes throughout the life span. There are genetic variants that help determine the length of the endogenous circadian cycle; a shorter length of the cycle may be associated with the early chronotype.[26] Prevalence of the late chronotype may be higher in men compared with women. The early chronotype is more prevalent in children, but with puberty this shifts to the late chronotype. Then in middle age, a shift back to the early type is observed.[26] The evening chronotype is associated with having excess weight and diabetes.[25]

Social jet lag is the misalignment between an individual's circadian system and their actual sleep and wake times due to social demands. This misalignment occurs due to the difference in sleep and wake demands imposed by schedules on workdays and the sleep and wake times based on preference during days off.[25] In a population-based cohort of the Dutch population, among individuals less than 61 years of age, social jet lag of greater than or equal to 2 hours was associated with increased risk of MetS (ATP III criteria) and diabetes/prediabetes (prevalence ratio and 95% CI: 2.13, 1.3 to 3.4 and 1.75, 1.2 to 2.5, respectively) after adjustment for sex, employment status, and education level.[27] Although MetS was not examined specifically, a study of 447 adults in the United States found social jet lag to be associated with greater insulin resistance and adiposity along with lower HDL, higher TGs, and higher fasting plasma insulin levels (all P values <.05).[25]

Lastly, shift work often involves sleeping during the day and eating during the night along with inadequate sleep duration, which dramatically alter the circadian system. With 15% of United States workforce engaged in work outside of traditional work hours, shift work is prevalent.[28] When eating late in the evening or in the middle of night, food intake occurs when circulating leptin levels, which help signal satiety, are lower than when eating at normal times or when in phase with biological clocks. This results in overeating of high-fat, calorie-dense foods, which impairs glucose tolerance and insulin sensitivity.[24] Misaligned sleep may alter the make-up of the gut microbiome whereas misaligned eating disturbs its rhythmic expression, which contributes to insulin resistance, inflammation, and adiposity.[24,29]

INSOMNIA AND METABOLIC SYNDROME

Insomnia is one of the most common sleep disorders and is characterized by sleep-specific complaints of difficulty falling asleep, difficulty staying asleep, or poor sleep quality despite adequate opportunity for sleep and impairments in daytime functioning. Prevalence rates of insomnia in the general population range from 4% to 48%, depending on the stringency of criteria used to define insomnia.[4] Insomnia can be chronic or acute, depending on the duration of sleep difficulties, and often is comorbid with medical and psychiatric disorders. Various risk factors for insomnia have been identified, including female sex, older age, ethnic minorities, minimal education, unemployment, depression, anxiety, substance use and abuse, and medical comorbidities.[30] Insomnia is associated with adverse physical and emotional health outcomes, including cardiometabolic disease, poor health-related quality of life, psychiatric disorders, workplace accidents and lost work productivity, and increased risk for all-cause mortality.[30]

Multiple cross-sectional studies have shown a significant relationship between insomnia and MetS. Zou and colleagues[31] assessed the relationship between insomnia and MetS (ATP III criteria) among 830 middle-aged (50–64 years old) adults from Sweden, in which 12.4% had insomnia defined by an Insomnia Severity Index score of greater than or equal to 15. Insomnia independently increased the risk of MetS (odds ratio [OR] 1.97; 95% CI, 1.00 to 3.86), even controlling for sleep duration and physician-diagnosed sleep apnea. Individuals with insomnia had lower HDL cholesterol and higher TGs than those without insomnia. Similarly, insomnia symptoms significantly increased the odds of having each component of MetS, including high waist circumference, low HDL, high low-density lipoprotein (LDL), high TGs, and high fasting plasma glucose level (IDF criteria) after controlling for sleep duration in a large sample (N = 26,016) of Taiwanese adults aged 35 years and older.[32]

A couple of cross-sectional studies have examined the relationship between specific insomnia symptoms (ie, difficulty initiating sleep, difficulty maintaining sleep, and early morning awakening) and MetS. In a population-based sample from Taiwan (N = 4197), difficulty initiating sleep (OR 1.24; 95% CI, 1.01 to 1.51) and difficulty maintaining sleep (OR 1.28; 95% CI, 1.02 to 1.61) were associated with the MetS (IDF and AHA/NHLBI criteria) after controlling for sleep duration.[33] Among an elderly community-dwelling population aged 65 years or older in France (N = 6354), difficulty maintaining sleep was independently associated with MetS (ATP III criteria) (OR 1.23; 95% CI, 1.06 to 1.43) and central obesity (OR 1.20; 95% CI, 1.06 to 1.36).[34]

Studies investigating sex and age differences in the relationship between insomnia and MetS have reported conflicting results. In a study of Chinese adults (N = 8017),[35] a significant association between insomnia and MetS (IDF criteria) was found only for men (OR 1.36; 95% CI, 1.02 to 1.77) and middle-aged (40–59 years) adults (OR 1.40; 95% CI, 1.09 to 1.79). There was no significant association between insomnia and MetS in women or in younger (<40 years) or older (≥60 years) adults. In a study of French adults (aged 18–65 years) with major depressive episode (N = 624),[10] severe insomnia increased the prevalence of MetS (ATP III criteria) (OR 2.2; 95% CI, 1.3 to 3.9) and IDF (OR 1.8; 95% CI, 1.1 to 2.9) definitions in women, not men. Furthermore, women aged over 50 years had a greater risk of MetS than those under 50 years. In a study of postmenopausal Ecuadorian women (N = 204; mean age 56 years),[36] however, insomnia was not significantly associated with the MetS (ATP III criteria) or its components.

Studies using a longitudinal design have estimated the risk of incident MetS associated with insomnia. Among a sample of 242 Italian police officers (mean age 36 years), insomnia at baseline significantly increased the risk for incidence of MetS (IDF and ATP III criteria) at 5-year follow-up after controlling for sleep duration, excessive daytime sleepiness, and sleep satisfaction (OR 11.04; 95% CI, 2.57 to 42.49).[37] More specifically, insomnia was associated with abdominal obesity (OR 5.83; 95% CI, 1.34 to 25.45) and low HDL cholesterol (OR 6.97; 95% CI, 1.06 to 45.99). In a study of Taiwanese older adults (aged 65 and older),[38] those with insomnia were more than 2 times more likely to have the MetS (ATP III criteria) at 1 year follow-up (OR 2.15; 95% CI, 1.09 to 4.22) after controlling for the components of MetS at baseline.

OBSTRUCTIVE SLEEP APNEA AND METABOLIC SYNDROME

OSA, the most common sleep-related breathing disorder, is characterized by repetitive occurrences of complete (apneas) or partial (hypopneas) upper airway obstruction during sleep that results in hypoxia and frequent arousals.[2] The apnea-hypopnea index (AHI) measures OSA severity and is calculated by dividing the total number of apneas and hypopneas by the total time of evaluated nasal airflow.[39] Commonly reported symptoms include breathing pauses during sleep, loud snoring, waking up choking or gasping for air, frequent awakenings, morning headaches, and excessive daytime sleepiness.[2]

Primary risk factors for OSA include central adiposity and the male sex. Women's rates of OSA increase during the menopause transition.[40] The risk for OSA increases with older age and greater weight gain and generally is more prevalent and severe among persons with morbid obesity.[41,42]

Although the different metabolic disorders in MetS have specific pathogenic pathways, in common is the visceral adiposity obesity phenotype.[43] As a result, there has been considerable research searching for a common link between OSA and visceral adiposity and their combined roles in MetS. Clinically, people with OSA may be more likely to gain weight and have difficulty losing it.[44] With OSA, recurrent obstructed breathing events result in repeated cycles of hypoxia-reoxygenation, with subsequent disruption of sleep throughout the night.[42] This may lead to stress-related neurohumoral activation and was shown in animals to be a potential mechanistic pathway for metabolic dysregulation in OSA.[42] The repeated cycles of hypoxia-reoxygenation affect different organs and adipose tissue, with dysfunctional adipose tissue playing an important role in the disposition toward development of MetS in persons with OSA.[42]

The coexistence of MetS, previously referred to as syndrome X, with OSA, sometimes referred to as syndrome Z,[45] has been supported in multiple studies. A study of 228 consecutive patients evaluated in a sleep clinic found that MetS (AHA/NHLBI criteria) coexisted in 60% of the 146 patients with OSA.[46] Another study in China (N = 178) of persons with severe OSA (AHI $\geq$30) found a significantly higher prevalence of coexisting MetS (ATP III criteria) in patients with excessive daytime sleepiness compared with those without sleepiness (78.2% vs 28.6%, respectively; $P<.001$).[47] Patients with severe OSA and excessive daytime sleepiness met more of the diagnostic criteria for MetS compared with those with severe OSA but without excessive daytime sleepiness (3.22 $\pm$ 0.94 vs 1.96 $\pm$ 1.06, respectively; $P<.001$).[47]

A meta-analysis examined the association between OSA and MetS parameters (ATP III criteria) in 10 studies (pooled total sample = 2053).[48] The analysis found that patients with OSA had significantly poorer values in MetS components (ie, higher systolic BP, lower HDL, and higher LDL) compared with those without OSA (all P values less than .001).

Recent evidence suggests that OSA and insomnia frequently coexist. Troxel and colleagues[49] longitudinally examined the relationship between sleep symptoms, including symptoms of insomnia and SDB and MetS (N = 812; United States adults aged 45–75 years; ATP III criteria). Difficulty initiating sleep, unrefreshing sleep, and loud snoring were significantly associated with an increased risk of developing the MetS over a 3-year follow-up period after controlling for demographics, lifestyle factors, and depressive symptoms. After further adjustment for AHI, however, only loud snoring remained a significant predictor of the incidence of MetS (OR 3.01; 95% CI, 1.39 to 6.55), whereas difficulty initiating sleep and unrefreshing sleep were reduced to nonsignificance. This may suggest that the MetS is more strongly associated with SDB than insomnia.

ASSESSMENT AND INTERVENTIONS TO IMPROVE SLEEP

Because sleep is an essential part of maintaining health, it should be part of the health provider's routine assessment in persons with MetS. This assessment should cover both factors that are integral for sleep health and signs/symptoms of common sleep disorders.[50] There are 5 dimensions that characterize sleep health that are important to evaluate as part of an assessment: satisfaction of sleep quality, alertness, timing of sleep, sleep efficiency, and sleep duration—or the acronym, SATED.[50] Because sleep disorders are prevalent in persons with MetS, it is especially important for health providers to ask focused questions to elicit information about symptoms of sleep disorders of insomnia, misalignment of circadian rhythms, and OSA. Responses that suggest a problem with sleep can be screened further with a validated instrument, which may suggest further evaluation by a specialist in sleep medicine.

There are validated self-report instruments to screen for potential sleep problems. One of the most widely used instruments to evaluate subjective sleepiness is the Epworth Sleepiness Scale,[51] an 8-question instrument that asks the likelihood of falling asleep in various circumstances with responses that range from "no likelihood of dozing or sleeping" to "strong likelihood of dozing or sleeping." Two questionnaires that can be used to evaluate the risk of OSA are the Berlin Questionnaire[52] and the STOP BANG.[53] The presence and severity of OSA requires an overnight sleep study that may be done either in laboratory or at home. Insomnia severity can be evaluated by use of the Insomnia Severity Index, a 7-item questionnaire that queries whether there is difficulty in falling asleep, maintaining sleep, or waking too early and whether these symptoms affect nighttime sleep quality or daytime functional ability.[54]

Many medications that treat components of MetS can negatively affect sleep because of worsened insomnia symptoms or because of increased weight gain and new or more severe OSA.[55] Therefore, health care providers are encouraged to carefully review whether all medications prescribed to patients with MetS do not have unintended effects on sleep (**Table 2**).

Sleep hygiene refers to routines and behaviors that are associated with good sleep (see Clinical Care Points). Components of good sleep hygiene include avoiding certain substances (ie, caffeine, nicotine, and alcohol) before bedtime and reducing stress.[56] Other sleep hygiene recommendations include minimizing noise, maintaining a regular schedule for bedtime and wake-up, allowing adequate time in bed to obtain 7 hours to 9 hours of sleep, and avoiding long naps (>30 minutes) or evening naps, especially if disruptive to being able to sleep at night. Although there is universal agreement on the importance of sleep hygiene, unfortunately, sleep hygiene recommendations have not, to the authors' knowledge, been evaluated on whether or not they directly improve MetS.

There have been interventions to improve total sleep time for short sleepers. Intervention feasibility and randomized control trial studies have looked at improvement of short sleep duration, but the findings are limited to sleep measures.[57] Results of a feasibility study that examined the effect of a personalized sleep extension protocol on nutrition found a reduction in consumption of free sugar but the study did not measure MetS component outcomes.[58] Several other studies focused on weight loss management programs (ie, nonsleep interventions) and have shown mixed results for improvement of total sleep time and metabolic outcomes.[59,60]

Table 2
Medications prescribed for metabolic syndrome conditions that affect sleep[55]

Indication	Classification	Example of Medications (Trade Names)	Effect on Sleep
Hypertension	β-Blockers	Metoprolol (Lopressor), atenolol (Tenormin), propranolol (Inderal)	Insomnia, night-time awakenings, nightmares
	α-Agonist	Clonidine (Catapres)	Daytime drowsiness and fatigue, disrupted rapid-eye-movement sleep, restlessness, early morning awakenings, nightmares
	α-Blockers	Tamsulosin (Flomax) Prazosin (Minipress)	Daytime drowsiness and fatigue, decreased rapid-eye-movement sleep
	Thiazide diuretics	Hydrochlorothiazide, chlorthalidone	Increased night-time urination, nocturnal leg cramps
	Angiotensin-converting enzyme inhibitors	Losartan (Cozaar) Valsartan (Diovan)	Disruptive cough and leg cramps
	Angiotensin receptor blockers	Losartan (Cozaar) Valsartan (Diovan)	Disruptive leg cramps, muscle aches
Cholesterol	Statins	Simvastatin (Zocor), atorvastatin (Lipitor)	Insomnia, disrupted sleep due to muscle pain
Hyperglycemic medications	Insulin, sulfonylureas	Insulin lispro (Humalog), glargine, glipizide, glyburide	Weight gain (OSA risk)
Obesity	Weight loss medications	Phentermine (Adipex-P), phentermine/ topiramate extended release (Qsymia), phendimetrazine (Bontril), bupropion/naltrexone (Contrave)	Insomnia symptoms, difficulty falling asleep or staying asleep

Numerous nonpharmacologic countermeasures to mitigate circadian misalignment and its metabolic consequences exist. Bright light exposure at the appropriate time and the avoidance of light at the wrong time are effective strategies to accelerate circadian rhythm entrainment. Individuals with a late chronotype or who are experiencing social jet lag might include bright light in the morning and blue light-blocking glasses or use applications on electronic devices to block short-wavelength emissions.[61,62] For shift workers, this would include a total 3 hours to 6 hours of bright light exposure during the night shift along with the avoidance of bright light during the commute home.[61]

Time-restricted eating, which limits eating to a 10-hour to 12-hour window, thus allowing for daily fasting of 12 hours or more, is an emerging countermeasure.[63] Because energy intake is a zeitgeber that has an impact on the circadian system, the proposed mechanism for time-restricted eating is to resynchronize the circadian-system with the external environment in situations where circadian misalignment may occur.[63] This resynchronization is hypothesized to help prevent or reverse MetS through pathways that influence glucose metabolism and inflammation.[64]

Behavioral sleep interventions should be done before considering the use of hypnotic medications in persons with complaints of insomnia.[3] Modifiable factors associated with insomnia need to be evaluated, such as medications, nocturia, and psychosocial factors. Persons with insomnia need to reduce their time in bed when not sleeping and to sleep when tired and ready to fall asleep. Things to be avoided are trying to fall asleep, daytime naps, clock watching, stimulants (eg, caffeine, tobacco, and prescribed medications that are intended for daytime), and alcohol as a sleep aid before bedtime.

Cognitive-behavior therapy for insomnia (CBT-I) is a behavioral treatment of chronic insomnia.[3,30] CBT-I focuses on addressing maladaptive behaviors and dysfunctional thoughts that perpetuate or exacerbate poor sleep quality and quantity and associate daytime impairments. The common therapeutic techniques of CBT-I include sleep restriction, stimulus control therapy, relaxation, cognitive therapies, mindfulness-based stress reduction, sleep hygiene education, and a combination of these techniques. The effect of CBT-I, however, has not been examined in persons with MetS. Given the close relationship between insomnia and MetS, the effect of CBT-I on MetS should be investigated further.

The gold standard for OSA treatment is continuous positive airway pressure (CPAP), a mask worn when sleeping in which a constant level of air pressure is continuously applied to the upper airway, but it sometimes is difficult to tolerate. Persons prescribed CPAP need to be encouraged to wear their devices every night for the entire night. If there is difficulty, communication with their health care provider may help problem-solve to improve adherence. For persons unable to tolerate CPAP, alternative treatments have arisen, such as hypoglossal nerve stimulation (a small device is surgically implanted in the chest stimulates a nerve that keeps the upper airway open), oral appliances that prevent the tongue from obstructive the upper airway, and behavioral modifications, such as weight loss.[42]

Various studies have not been able to establish that treatment of OSA consistently is associated with improvements in the metabolic components of obesity, insulin-glucose dysmetabolism, dyslipidemia, or systemic inflammation.[65,66] Studies have been conflicting regarding weight loss and CPAP treatment. A recent meta-analysis suggests CPAP treatment may lead to increased weight unless patients are counseled to be proactive in not gaining weight.[67]

SUMMARY

This article reviews evidence on relationships between sleep disorders and the development and severity of MetS and discusses effective interventions for sleep and MetS. Multiple studies report a U-shaped association between persons with normal sleep duration and approximately 7 hours sleep per night showed the lowest risk for MetS. Insomnia independently increases the risk of MetS in various populations; however, some studies have shown inconsistent findings across age and gender. Although there is limited research on circadian misalignment with individuals with MetS, circadian misalignment is associated with impaired glucose control and increased inflammatory markers, resulting in increased risk for cardiometabolic conditions. OSA and MetS are strongly associated. Multiple studies corroborate that visceral obesity as a component of Mets may contribute to increased risk for OSA. Excessive daytime sleepiness in the presence of OSA may contribute to worse MetS outcomes. Effective interventions to improve sleep include good sleep hygiene, weight loss programs, restricted eating time and sugar consumption, CBT-I, and CPAP for individuals with OSA. Based on significant relationships between sleep disorders and MetS, interventions to significantly improve sleep would have potential to affect MetS positively.

CLINICS CARE POINTS

- Evaluation of obesity needs to consider weight distribution because central adiposity is a hallmark of both MetS and OSA.

- Persons with MetS and any sleep problem should be encouraged to improve their basic sleep hygiene behaviors.

- Exercise should be encouraged to promote good sleep during the day.

- Persons should avoid stimulating substances (ie, caffeine, nicotine, and prescribed medications that worsen sleep) close to bedtime.

- Sleep duration for adults and older adults is recommended to be between 7 hours and 9 hours a night.

- Persons with MetS need to be evaluated during their routine visits by their health care provider, whether they snore or hold their breath while sleeping.

- Adherence to treatment with CPAP, if appropriate, is encouraged. Conventional medical approaches to OSA treatment, including positional treatment, avoidance of alcohol, and weight loss, also can be incorporated.

- Persons with unintended microsleeps (ie, falling asleep even briefly) should be evaluated for sleep disorders. This is true especially if sleep attacks occur during situations that require vigilance, for example, driving a car.

- Maintaining a regular sleep routine promotes sleep health. Bedtime should be before midnight on most nights and wake time should stay constant, even if it is difficult to fall asleep.

- Women with obesity, at the menopausal transition, or who complain of insomnia, fatigue, or depression should be evaluated for SDB.

DISCLOSURE

C. Godzik has a National Institute of Mental Health (NIMH) Postdoctoral Research Fellowship in Geriatric Mental Health Services (5 T32 MH 073553) and J. Kariuki has a Diversity Supplement grant from the National Heart, Lung, and Blood Institute (NHLBI, R01 HL131583S). All other authors have nothing to disclose.

REFERENCES

1. World Health Organization. Constitution. Available at: https://www.who.int/about/who-we-are/constitution. Accessed October 1, 2020.
2. Lee W, Nagubadi S, Kryger MH, et al. Epidemiology of obstructive sleep apnea: A population-based perspective. Expert Rev Respir Med 2008;2(3):349–64.
3. Buysse DJ. Insomnia. JAMA 2013;309(7):706–16.

4. Ohayon MM. Epidemiology of insomnia: What we know and what we still need to learn. Sleep Med Rev 2002;6(2):97–111.
5. Hirode G, Wong RJ. Trends in the prevalence of metabolic syndrome in the United States, 2011-2016. JAMA 2020;323(24):2526–8.
6. Moore JX, Chaudhary N, Akinyemiju T. Metabolic syndrome prevalence by race/ethnicity and sex in the United States, National Health and Nutrition Examination Survey, 1988-2012. Prev Chronic Dis 2017;14:E24.
7. Ogden CL, Fryar CD, Martin CB, et al. Trends in obesity prevalence by race and Hispanic origin-1999-2000 to 2017-2018. JAMA 2020;324(12):1208–10.
8. Desroches S, Lamarche B. The evolving definitions and increasing prevalence of the metabolic syndrome. Appl Physiol Nutr Metab 2007;32(1):23–32.
9. Grundy SM, Cleeman JI, Daniels SR, et al. Diagnosis and management of the metabolic syndrome: An American Heart Association/National Heart, Lung, and Blood Institute Scientific Statement. Circulation 2005;112(17):2735–52.
10. Costemale-Lacoste JF, Asmar KE, Rigal A, et al. Severe insomnia is associated with metabolic syndrome in women over 50 years with major depression treated in psychiatry settings: a METADAP report. J Affect Disord 2020;264:513–8.
11. Lloyd-Jones DM. Cardiovascular risk prediction: Basic concepts, current status, and future directions. Circulation 2010;121(15):1768–77.
12. O'Neill S, O'Driscoll L. Metabolic syndrome: A closer look at the growing epidemic and its associated pathologies. Obes Rev 2015;16(1):1–12.
13. Ervin RB. Prevalence of metabolic syndrome among adults 20 years of age and over, by sex, age, race and ethnicity, and body mass index: United States, 2003-2006. Natl Health Stat Rep 2009;(13):1–7.
14. Obunai K, Jani S, Dangas GD. Cardiovascular morbidity and mortality of the metabolic syndrome. Med Clin North Am 2007;91(6):1169–84, x.
15. Lopez-Candales A, Hernandez Burgos PM, Hernandez-Suarez DF, et al. Linking chronic inflammation with cardiovascular disease: From normal aging to the metabolic syndrome. J Nat Sci 2017;3(4):e341.
16. Hirshkowitz M, Whiton K, Albert SM, et al. National Sleep Foundation's sleep time duration recommendations: Methodology and results summary. Sleep Health 2015;1(1):40–3.
17. Matsumoto T, Chin K. Prevalence of sleep disturbances: Sleep disordered breathing, short sleep duration, and non-restorative sleep. Respir Investig 2019;57(3):227–37.
18. Stamatakis KA, Punjabi NM. Long sleep duration: A risk to health or a marker of risk? Sleep Med Rev 2007;11(5):337–9.
19. Luyster FS, Baniak LM, Chasens ER, et al. Sleep among working adults. In: Duncan DT, Kawachi I, Redline S, editors. Social epidemiology of sleep. Oxford (United Kingdom): Oxford University Press; 2019. p. 119–38.
20. Whinnery J, Jackson N, Rattanaumpawan P, et al. Short and long sleep duration associated with race/ethnicity, sociodemographics, and socioeconomic position. Sleep 2014;37(3):601–11.
21. Cappuccio FP, Cooper D, D'Elia L, et al. Sleep duration predicts cardiovascular outcomes: A systematic review and meta-analysis of prospective studies. Eur Heart J 2011;32(12):1484–92.
22. Smiley A, King D, Bidulescu A. The association between sleep duration and metabolic syndrome: The NHANES 2013/2014. Nutrients 2019;11(11):2582.
23. Anothaisintawee T, Lertrattananon D, Thamakaison S, et al. Later chronotype is associated with higher hemoglobin A1c in prediabetes patients. Chronobiol Int 2017;34(3):393–402.

24. James SM, Honn KA, Gaddameedhi S, et al. Shift work: Disrupted circadian rhythms and sleep-implications for health and well-being. Curr Sleep Med Rep 2017;3(2):104–12.
25. Wong PM, Hasler BP, Kamarck TW, et al. Social jetlag, chronotype, and cardio-metabolic risk. J Clin Endocrinol Metab 2015;100(12):4612–20.
26. Almoosawi S, Vingeliene S, Gachon F, et al. Chronotype: Implications for epide-miologic studies on chrono-nutrition and cardiometabolic health. Adv Nutr 2019; 10(1):30–42.
27. Koopman ADM, Rauh SP, van 't Riet E, et al. The association between social jet-lag, the metabolic syndrome, and type 2 diabetes mellitus in the general popula-tion: The New Hoorn Study. J Biol Rhythms 2017;32(4):359–68.
28. Wright KP Jr, Bogan RK, Wyatt JK. Shift work and the assessment and manage-ment of shift work disorder (SWD). Sleep Med Rev 2013;17(1):41–54.
29. Bae SA, Fang MZ, Rustgi V, et al. At the interface of lifestyle, behavior, and circa-dian rhythms: Metabolic implications. Front Nutr 2019;6:132.
30. Lichstein KL, Taylor DJ, McCrae CS, et al. Insomnia: Epidemiology and risk fac-tors. In: Kryger M, Roth T, Dement WC, editors. Principles and practice of sleep medicine. Philadelphia: Saunders/Elsevier; 2017. p. 761–8.
31. Zou D, Wennman H, Hedner J, et al. Insomnia is associated with metabolic syn-drome in a middle-aged population: the SCAPIS pilot cohort. Eur J Prev Cardiol 2020;2047487320940862.
32. Syauqy A, Hsu CY, Rau HH, et al. Association of sleep duration and insomnia symptoms with components of metabolic syndrome and inflammation in middle-aged and older adults with metabolic syndrome in Taiwan. Nutrients 2019;11(8):1848.
33. Lin SC, Sun CA, You SL, et al. The link of self-reported insomnia symptoms and sleep duration with metabolic syndrome: A Chinese population-based study. Sleep 2016;39(6):1261–6.
34. Akbaraly TN, Jaussent I, Besset A, et al. Sleep complaints and metabolic syn-drome in an elderly population: The Three-City Study. Am J Geriatr Psychiatry 2015;23(8):818–28.
35. Wang Y, Jiang T, Wang X, et al. Association between insomnia and metabolic syn-drome in a Chinese Han population: A Cross-sectional Study. Sci Rep 2017;7(1): 10893.
36. Chedraui P, San Miguel G, Villacreses D, et al. Assessment of insomnia and related risk factors in postmenopausal women screened for the metabolic syn-drome. Maturitas 2013;74(2):154–9.
37. Garbarino S, Magnavita N. Sleep problems are a strong predictor of stress-related metabolic changes in police officers. A prospective study. PLoS One 2019;14(10):e0224259.
38. Chen LJ, Lai YJ, Sun WJ, et al. Associations of exercise, sedentary time and insomnia with metabolic syndrome in Taiwanese older adults: A 1-year follow-up study. Endocr Res 2015;40(4):220–6.
39. Kapur VK, Auckley DH, Chowdhuri S, et al. Clinical practice guideline for diag-nostic testing for adult obstructive sleep apnea: An American Academy of Sleep Medicine Clinical Practice Guideline. J Clin Sleep Med 2017;13(3):479–504.
40. Redline S. Obstructive sleep apnea: Phenotypes and genetics. In: Kryger TR MH, Dement WC, editors. Principles and practice of geriatric sleep medicine. 6th edi-tion. Philadelphia: Elsevier; 2017. p. 1102–9.
41. Jehan S, Zizi F, Pandi-Perumal SR, et al. Obstructive sleep apnea and obesity: Implications for public health. Sleep Med Disord 2017;1(4):00019.

42. Sau-Man Ip M. Obstructive sleep apnea and metabolic disorders. In: Kryger TR MH, Dement WC, editors. Principles and practice of sleep medicine. 6th edition. Philadelphia: Elsevier; 2017. p. 1167–8.

43. Ritchie SA, Connell JM. The link between abdominal obesity, metabolic syndrome and cardiovascular disease. Nutr Metab Cardiovasc Dis 2007;17(4):319–26.

44. Kline CE, Burke LE, Sereika SM, et al. Bidirectional relationships between weight change and sleep apnea in a behavioral weight loss intervention. Mayo Clin Proc 2018;93(9):1290–8.

45. Wilcox I, McNamara SG, Collins FL, et al. Syndrome Z": The interaction of sleep apnoea, vascular risk factors and heart disease. Thorax 1998;53(Suppl 3):S25–8.

46. Parish JM, Adam T, Facchiano L. Relationship of metabolic syndrome and obstructive sleep apnea. J Clin Sleep Med 2007;3(5):467–72.

47. Huang JF, Chen LD, Lin QC, et al. The relationship between excessive daytime sleepiness and metabolic syndrome in severe obstructive sleep apnea syndrome. Clin Respir J 2016;10(6):714–21.

48. Kong DL, Qin Z, Wang W, et al. Association between obstructive sleep apnea and metabolic syndrome: A meta-analysis. Clin Invest Med 2016;39(5):E161–72.

49. Troxel WM, Buysse DJ, Matthews KA, et al. Sleep symptoms predict the development of the metabolic syndrome. Sleep 2010;33(12):1633–40.

50. Buysse DJ. Sleep health: can we define it? Does it matter? Sleep 2014; 37(1):9–17.

51. Johns MW. A new method for measuring daytime sleepiness: The Epworth Sleepiness Scale. Sleep 1991;14(6):540–5.

52. Netzer NC, Stoohs RA, Netzer CM, et al. Using the Berlin Questionnaire to identify patients at risk for the sleep apnea syndrome. Ann Intern Med 1999;131(7): 485–91.

53. Chung F, Abdullah HR, Liao P. STOP-Bang Questionnaire: A practical approach to screen for obstructive sleep apnea. Chest 2016;149(3):631–8.

54. Bastien CH, Vallieres A, Morin CM. Validation of the Insomnia Severity Index as an outcome measure for insomnia research. Sleep Med 2001;2(4):297–307.

55. Harvard News Letter. Medications that can affect sleep. Harvard Health Publishing. 2020. Available at: https://www.health.harvard.edu/newsletter_article/medications-that-can-affect-sleep. Accessed October 6, 2020.

56. Irish LA, Kline CE, Gunn HE, et al. The role of sleep hygiene in promoting public health: A review of empirical evidence. Sleep Med Rev 2015;22:23–36.

57. Cheikh M, Hammouda O, Gaamouri N, et al. Melatonin ingestion after exhaustive late-evening exercise improves sleep quality and quantity, and short-term performances in teenage athletes. Chronobiol Int 2018;35(9):1281–93.

58. Al Khatib HK, Hall WL, Creedon A, et al. Sleep extension is a feasible lifestyle intervention in free-living adults who are habitually short sleepers: a potential strategy for decreasing intake of free sugars? A randomized controlled pilot study. Am J Clin Nutr 2018;107(1):43–53.

59. Chang MW, Tan A, Schaffir J, et al. Sleep and weight loss in low-income overweight or obese postpartum women. BMC Obes 2019;6:12.

60. Goerke M, Sobieray U, Becke A, et al. Successful physical exercise-induced weight loss is modulated by habitual sleep duration in the elderly: results of a pilot study. J Neural Transm (Vienna) 2017;124(Suppl 1):153–62.

61. Dodson ER, Zee PC. Therapeutics for Circadian Rhythm Sleep Disorders. Sleep Med Clin 2010;5(4):701–15.

62. Potter GD, Skene DJ, Arendt J, et al. Circadian Rhythm and Sleep Disruption: Causes, Metabolic Consequences, and Countermeasures. Endocr Rev 2016; 37(6):584–608.
63. Chaix A, Manoogian ENC, Melkani GC, et al. Time-Restricted Eating to Prevent and Manage Chronic Metabolic Diseases. Annu Rev Nutr 2019;39:291–315.
64. Longo VD, Panda S. Fasting, Circadian Rhythms, and Time-Restricted Feeding in Healthy Lifespan. Cell Metab 2016;23(6):1048–59.
65. Jullian-Desayes I, Joyeux-Faure M, Tamisier R, et al. Impact of obstructive sleep apnea treatment by continuous positive airway pressure on cardiometabolic biomarkers: a systematic review from sham CPAP randomized controlled trials. Sleep Med Rev 2015;21:23–38.
66. Schlatzer C, Schwarz EI, Kohler M. The effect of continuous positive airway pressure on metabolic variables in patients with obstructive sleep apnoea. Chron Respir Dis 2014;11(1):41–52.
67. Drager LF, Brunoni AR, Jenner R, et al. Effects of CPAP on body weight in patients with obstructive sleep apnoea: A meta-analysis of randomized trials. Thorax 2015;70(3):258–64.

Sleep and Mental Health

Understanding and Addressing the Unique Challenges and Conditions of the Veteran: Improving Sleep and Well-Being

Sandra Estes, EdD, MSN[a,b,*],
Johnny R. Tice, DNP, MA, CRNP, FNP-C, PMHNP-BC[a]

KEYWORDS

- Sleep • Veteran • Mental health • Substance use • Primary care

KEY POINTS

- Veterans present unique challenges for clinicians treating sleep disorders and substance use in the primary care setting.
- All health care clinicians should have easy and accessible resources for the care of veterans.
- Sleep problems can coexist and exacerbate mental illness, and treatment of substance use disorders may interfere with sleep quality.
- Interprofessional collaboration improves veteran health outcomes and enhances clinician professional development.

 Video content accompanies this article at http://www.nursing.theclinics.com

INTRODUCTION

Originally established after World War I, the Veterans Administration (VA) was built to provide health care for conditions related to their military experiences. In 1989, the veterans' health care system was transformed and renamed Veterans Health Administration (VHA). The VHA missions included providing medical care for eligible veterans; training health care professionals; conducting research; providing contingency support to the military health care system and national disaster assistance; and serving

[a] Capstone College of Nursing, The University of Alabama, 650 University Boulevard East, Tuscaloosa, AL 35401, USA; [b] Tuscaloosa Veterans Affairs Medical Center, Tuscaloosa Research and Education Advancement Corporation, 3701 Loop Road East, Building 3 Research Suite, Tuscaloosa, AL 35404, USA
* Corresponding author. Capstone College of Nursing, The University of Alabama, Box 870358, Tuscaloosa, AL 35486-0358.
E-mail address: sestes@ua.edu

Nurs Clin N Am 56 (2021) 219–227
https://doi.org/10.1016/j.cnur.2021.03.002
0029-6465/21/© 2021 Elsevier Inc. All rights reserved.

nursing.theclinics.com

the homeless.[1] The VHA facilities offer treatment for all or most of the health care needs of its veterans. According to VHA transition assistance program, nearly 200,000 services members transition to civilian life every year, directly contributing to the total number of veterans, which is roughly 18,000,000 (5.5% of the nation's population).[2-4] As of 2017, 49% of veterans present to a VHA facility to seek medical treatment.[5] Over the years, with the growing number of veterans, the wait list for assessment and treatments also grew. The VHA system found itself unable to keep up with the overwhelming demands and federal policy was written to expedite health care access and delivery to veterans in the Mission Act of 2018.[6] The Mission Act expanded veteran health care access allowing veterans to be seen and treated in civilian, non-VHA facilities. Although the VHA is the largest integrated health care system in the nation, providing many health care services and resources for these individuals, it is important for all health care clinicians to have an understanding of the unique challenges and conditions these individuals face and have the resources available to meet their health care needs.

SLEEP DISORDERS

The National Sleep Foundation (2015) recommends that adults from the age of 18 to 64 sleep between 7 and 9 hours each night; however, the Centers for Disease Control and Prevention reports nearly a third of the US adult population do not met this standard.[7,8] Only 25% to 35% of veterans attain the recommended 7 to 9 hours of sleep each night.[9] Sleep disorders are characterized by difficulty falling asleep, staying asleep, frequent awakenings, and/or prolonged sleep.[10] It is recognized and well documented that veterans have a high incidence and prevalence of homelessness, posttraumatic stress disorder (PTSD), and substance use disorder (SUD).[11,12] An increase in sleep disorders among veterans is also contributed to aging of the population and high rates of comorbidities.[9] Unfortunately, poor sleep habits for military personnel can exists for several years during service, and the effects of poor sleep may be more apparent during civilian life.

Homelessness

Evidence suggests that environmental factors can affect sleep.[13] In 2009, The National Center on Homelessness among Veterans, was created to promote research into the cause of homelessness among veterans and to identify and disseminate best practices for veterans at risk for or experiencing homelessness.[14] In 2012, the VHA incorporated a 2-question Homelessness Screening Clinical Reminder (HSCR) into the electronic medical record to identify veterans experiencing housing instability and to ensure referral to appropriate services when they are seen in VHA outpatient clinics.[15] Since that time, research on the use of HSCR among veterans has led to the recommendation for use in primary care settings in addition to the VHA.[16] For veterans who use the VHA, the HSCR is administered at least annually during outpatient visits to those not already receiving VA housing support services.

Screening: homelessness screening clinical reminder screening questions

1. In the past 2 months, have you been living in stable housing that you own, rent, or stay in as part of a household? (A negative response indicates housing instability.)
2. Are you worried or concerned that in the next 2 months you may not have stable housing that you own, rent, or stay in as part of a household? (A positive response indicates risk.)

Using this screening tool can serve as the foundation for capturing housing insta-bility and risk for housing instability and homelessness.[15] Understanding the relation-ship between homelessness and sleep disorders is important for the veteran's well-being. In general, people experiencing homelessness have high rates of severe mental illness. For some homeless veterans, the combination of mental illness and sleep deprivation can make it difficult to overcome situations surrounding homeless-ness.[17] Poor sleep for homeless individuals especially veterans, is precipitated many times by circumstantial proceedings such as exposure to extreme weather variability, self-guarding to prevent theft or assault, noise, lighting, lack of comfort, and hunger. Similar environmental factors affect veterans in homeless shelters in addition to over-crowding and lack of privacy.[17,18] Homeless veterans may be more likely to report less sleep, increased daytime sleepiness, and greater use of substances to stay awake during the day or aid in falling asleep.[17]

Referral

Veterans who are identified as having housing instability or risk of housing instability or homelessness should be connected as soon as possible to the National Center for Homelessness among Veterans. The National Call Center can be reached 24 hours a day, 7 days a week via phone at 877-4AID-VET (877-424-3838) or chat online at va.gov/homeless. A trained VA staff member will ask a few questions and connect you with a local VA specialist who can help with homeless programs and services.[19]

Posttraumatic Stress Disorder

PTSD occurs when an individual is exposed to death, threatened death, actual or threatened serious injury, or actual or threatened sexual violence.[20] Through their ser-vice, including combat missions, many veterans met criteria and suffer with the asso-ciated symptoms and experiences including flashbacks, nightmares, and intrusive thoughts.[21] When an individual is continuously battling symptoms related to traumatic event(s), their overall well-being is compromised and, in many cases, this also affects their overall sleep and sleep quality.

Sleep disturbance is found in 90% to 100% of veterans with PTSD.[22] When a sleep disorder co-occurs with PTSD in a veteran, it is important to assess whether the sleep disorder pre-dates the PTSD exposure and onset. In addition, sleep disorders should be assessed independently with respect to underlying etiologies such as medical, di-etary, and environmental.[23] If the co-occurring sleep disorder is insomnia, Cognitive Behavioral Therapy for Insomnia (CBT-I) is considered first-line treatment intervention with medication used as second-line treatment intervention.[24–26]

Screening

Clinicians may find the Primary Care PTSD Screen for DSM-5 (PC-PTSD-5)[21] (Appendix A), an easy to use, public domain, evidence-based tool that uses a 5-item screen to identify individuals who may have PTSD highly useful. A positive, or "yes" to 3 of the 5 questions indicates high probability of PTSD, which is valuable in identifying these individuals and initiating the appropriate interventions.

Treatment

Once a veteran meets criteria for PTSD using the DSM-5 criteria, the primary provider should use the treatment approach set forth by the VHA and Department of Defense (DoD) (Appendix B).[24] Main-stay treatment is focused on using trauma-focused psy-chotherapies.[27] If trauma-focused psychotherapies are not available, then non–trauma-focused psychotherapies are suggested and/or pharmacologic treatment as monotherapy or as augmentation to partial responders to psychotherapy.[24]

Case study
Appendix C is an author-generated case study of a 53-year-old veteran with sleep disturbance and PTSD. The case study is presented in SOAP (subjective, objective, assessment, and plan) format with evidence-based interventions for managing coexisting sleep disturbance and PTSD.

CBT-I uses behavior and cognitive approaches to improve insomnia and fatigue. Behavioral approaches can include muscle relaxation, sleep restriction, stimulus control, and sleep hygiene techniques. Cognitive approaches include patient self-monitoring of maladaptive cognitions such as catastrophic thinking.[28] El-Solh and colleagues[25] found when medication is used as a first-line treatment, it would negatively affect the efficacy of CBT-I. Favorable outcomes have been demonstrated for both active military and older veterans with CBT-I for sleep-related issues.[29,30] Patients prefer the convenience of having a multitude of CBT-I delivery options.[26] Koffel and colleagues[26] recently demonstrated that patients initially would attempt to manage their insomnia and fatigue symptoms using the CBT-I educational material such as books and Web-based programs, but would then proceed to provider-delivered CBT-I, if needed.

Telehealth services for sleep is another approach to improving sleep for the growing veteran population, and it is designed to improve accessibility for veterans in rural areas. Of the 9.1 million veterans currently enrolled in the VHA health care system, 2.8 million veterans live in rural or remote regions of the country. The TeleSleep Program has been introduced at the VHA and their associated community-based outpatient clinics. The synchronous telehealth service includes video conferencing between patient and providers. The asynchronous telehealth service enables non–sleep specialty providers (eg, mental health) to administer sleep studies and upload the data for sleep specialist to view and make recommendations. The e-consultation option can be used by non–sleep specialty providers to request a medical record review by the sleep specialist. Instead of the veteran waiting several weeks to months for an initial appointment, the sleep specialist can order the diagnostic sleep test and start treatment based on the test results. The use of innovative technologies can promote early detection of sleep disorders in veterans with psychological comorbidities such as PTSD and SUD.[9,31]

Substance Use Disorder

SUD is problematic and involves the use of 1 or more substances that results in impairment in daily function and psychological distress.[32] The Substance Abuse and Mental Health Services Administration[33] found substance use more common in veterans with mental illnesses and emphasizes the need to screen for all substances as well as mental disorders for all clinical evaluations. It is known that veterans are exposed to many combat exposures and stressors and a unique military culture that is much different from that of civilian life, increasing their overall risk for SUD.[34] For veterans who are first-time care users of the VHA system, nearly 11% meet criteria for SUD and approximately 1 in 10 veterans are diagnosed with an SUD, which is higher than that of the general population.[35]

Screening
Screening for SUDs should always use DSM-5 criteria to diagnose the disorder. SUD can include abuse of alcohol (ETOH), central nervous system (CNS) depressants (such as benzodiazepines), opioid use disorder (OUD), cannabis use disorder (CUD), tobacco, and stimulant use disorder.[36] Different tools that screen for alcohol use or illicit drug use such as Audit-C or ASSIST have been used to screen veterans for SUD.[37]

The Substance Use Brief Screen (SUBS), a relatively new tool, screens for unhealthy use of tobacco, alcohol, illicit drugs, and prescription drugs in a 4-question format taking approximately 1 to 2 minutes, saving valuable clinic time (Appendix D).[38] Using a more holistic approach, such as the SUBS tool, allows the clinician to capture the use of multiple substances leading to a more optimal course or courses of treatment and interventions. The positive correlations between insomnia and alcohol use in veterans have long been established.[39,40] In particular, the intrusive symptoms of PTSD have a positive correlation to both sleep and alcohol problems.[39] Women in particular are at a higher risk of using alcohol to self-medicate PTSD and insomnia symptoms.[40] Hoggatt and colleagues[41] caution that clinicians should use gender-tailored questions, such as the question used in the SUBS tool, to detect unhealthy alcohol use in women that would otherwise go unnoticed, such as with use of the AUDIT-C.

Treatment
All treatment interventions that follow were taken from the Department of Veterans Affairs guidelines and recommendations.[42]

Alcohol
The primary provider should use the treatment guidelines set forth by the VHA and DoD. These guidelines recommend medically supervised withdrawal management (usually inpatient) for individuals experiencing acute withdrawal to alcohol or CNS depressants who score $\geq$20 on the Clinical Institute Withdrawal Assessment for Alcohol (CIWA-Ar) (Appendix E).[42] These individuals require the use of stabilization of withdrawal symptoms using a predetermined amount of benzodiazepines and phenobarbital for replacement therapy and a tapering schedule based on CIWA-Ar scores. If these medications are contraindicated, alternative pharmacotherapy can include carbamazepine, gabapentin, or valproic acid as an alternative. Pharmacotherapies used for withdrawal and stabilization include naltrexone, acamprosate, disulfiram, topiramate, or gabapentin.

Opioids
Individuals with OUD are recommended to be prescribed a detoxification with long-term opioid agonists, such as methadone, buprenorphine, naltrexone, or other symptom-treatment medications for short-term, medically supervised withdrawal. If these treatments are contraindicated, clonidine as a second-line agent can be used to manage withdrawal symptoms. Once acute withdrawal has improved, maintenance therapy can include the same pharmacotherapy interventions used with short-term withdrawal.

Stimulant use disorder
There is insufficient evidence to make recommendations for or against the use of any pharmacotherapy to treat cocaine or methamphetamine use disorder. Withdrawal focuses on managing symptoms associated with acute intoxication and particular symptoms are treated as they manifest.

Cannabis use disorder
Evidence-based practice indicates insufficient evidence to recommend for or against pharmacotherapy for the treatment of CUD. However, there have been effective outcomes when treated with psychosocial interventions.

SUMMARY

In an effort to improve access to care for veterans, the Mission Act of 2018 allowed veterans to be treated in civilian, non-VHA facilities.[6] Many primary care providers in the civilian setting lack training related to the unique and specific challenges veterans face. More veterans are now being treated within the community setting than ever before, offering opportunities for community health care clinicians to enhance their skills set providing holistic care for this diverse population.

This article set out to offer primary care providers practicing in demanding settings a convenient way to access the guidelines that are used for providers who are trained to treat this particular population. These guidelines were crafted carefully and researched in a joint effort between the VHA and DoD to offer best practices for providers.

Screening tools were suggested in the assessment of homelessness, PTSD, and SUD. Treatment algorithms and referral sources were provided for acute and maintenance of these challenges. Finally, outcome evaluation, referrals, and follow-up strategies also were recommended.

CRITICS CARE POINTS

- Evidence-based sleep screening tools (eg, the Insomnia Severity Index) can be used in the primary care setting to examine sleep health among veterans.
- Treatment of PTSD with first-line pharmacologic treatment of antidepressants directly enhances sleep by increasing serotonin.
- CBT-I has been shown to be effective in managing sleep problems among veterans with SUD.
- Sleep disorders, if left untreated, may increase risk for relapse among veterans with SUD and mental illness
- During substance use treatment, some veterans may experience worse sleep associated with withdrawal symptoms.
- Poor sleep could also indicate relapse during the course of treatment for SUDs.
- Routine sleep assessments are important for all veterans and especially important for those with coexisting mental health disorders.

DISCLOSURE

The authors have nothing to disclose.

SUPPLEMENTARY DATA

Supplementary data related to this article can be found online at https://doi.org/10.1016/j.cnur.2021.03.002.

REFERENCES

1. Kizer KW, Dudley RA. Extreme makeover: transformation of the veterans health care system. Annu Rev Public Health 2009;30:313–39.
2. US Census Bureau. Quick facts United States 2019. Available at: https://www.census.gov/quickfacts/fact/table/US/PST045219. Accessed October 15,2020.
3. US Department of Veterans Affairs. Transition and economic development 2020. Available at: https://benefits.va.gov/transition/tap.asp. Accessed October 15, 2020.
4. US Census Bureau. Those who served: America's veterans from World War II to the War on Terror. American Community Survey; 2020. Available at: https://www.

census.gov/content/dam/Census/library/publications/2020/demo/acs-43.pdf. Accessed October 15,2020.

5. Maiocco G, Vance B, Dichiacchio T. Readiness of non-veteran health administration advanced practice registered nurses to care for those who have served: a multimethod descriptive study. Pol Polit Nurs Pract 2020;21(2):82–94.

6. The US Congress. VA Mission Act of 2018. 2018. Available at: https://www.congress.gov/115/bills/s2372/BILLS-115s2372enr.pdf. Accessed October 15, 2020.

7. Hirshkowitz M, Whiton K, Albert SM, et al. National Sleep Foundation's sleep time duration recommendations: methodology and results summary. Sleep Health 2015;1(1):40–3.

8. Centers for Disease Control and Prevention. Sleep and sleep disorders 2020. Available at: https://www.cdc.gov/sleep/index.html. Accessed October 15, 2020.

9. Sarmiento KF, Folmer RL, Stepnowsky CJ, et al. National expansion of sleep telemedicine for Veterans: The TeleSleep Program. J Clin Sleep Med 2019;15(9): 1355–64.

10. American Academy of Sleep Medicine. The international classification of sleep disorders – third edition (ICSD-3) 2014. Darien, IL.

11. Livingston N, Mahoney C, Ameral V, et al. Changes in alcohol use, PTSD hyperarousal symptoms, and intervention dropout following veterans use of VetChange. Addict Behav 2020;107:106401.

12. Tsai J, Rosenheck R. Risk factors for homelessness among US Veterans. Epidemiol Rev 2015;37:177–95.

13. Lewis V, Creamer M, Failla S. Is poor sleep in veterans a function of posttraumatic stress disorder? Mil Med 2009;174(9):948–51.

14. US Department of Veterans Affairs. Background on VHA's national center on homelessness among veterans 2019. Available at: https://www.va.gov/homeless/nchav/about-us/background.asp. Accessed October 15, 2020.

15. Montgomery A, Fargo J, Byrne T, et al. Universal screening for homelessness and risk for homelessness in the Veterans Health Administration. Am J Public Health 2013;103(2):210–1.

16. Chhabra M, Sorrentino AE, Cusack M, et al. Screening for housing instability: providers' reflections on addressing a social determinant of health. J Gen Intern Med 2019;3:1213–9.

17. Gonzalez A, Tyminski Q. Sleep deprivation in an American homeless population. Sleep health 2019;6(4):489–94.

18. De Fine Licht KP, Praksis EI. Hostile urban architecture: a critical discussion of the seemingly offensive art of keeping people away. Nordic J Appl Ethics 2017;11(2): 27–44.

19. US Department of Veterans Affairs. National call center for homeless veterans 2019. Available at: https://www.va.gov/homeless/nationalcallcenter.asp. Accessed October 15, 2020.

20. American Psychiatric Association. Diagnostic and Statistical Manual of Mental Disorders, Fifth Edition. Arlington (VA): American Psychiatric Association; 2013.

21. Wall PH, Convoy SP, Braybrook CJ. Military service-related post-traumatic stress disorder: Finding a way home. Nurs Clin North Am 2019;54:503–15.

22. Department of Veterans Affairs and Department of Defense. Clinical practice guideline for the management of posttraumatic stress disorder and acute stress disorder clinician summary. 2017. Washington, DC. Available at: https://www.healthquality.va.gov/guidelines/MH/ptsd/VADoDPTSDCPGClinicianSummary Final.pdf. Accessed October 15, 2020.

23. Youngren W, Miller K, Davis J. An assessment of medical practitioners knowledge of, experience with, and treatment attitudes towards sleep disorders and nightmares. J Clin Psychol Med Settings 2019;26:166–72.

24. Department of Veterans Affairs and Department of Defense. Clinical practice guideline for the management of posttraumatic stress disorder and acute stress disorder. 2017. Washington, DC. Available at: www.healthquality.va.gov/guidelines/MH/ptsd/VADoDPTSDCPGFinal.pdf. Accessed October 15, 2020.

25. El-Solh A, O'Brien N, Akinnusi M, et al. Predictors of cognitive behavioral therapy outcomes for insomnia in veterans with post-traumatic stress disorder. Sleep Breath 2019;23:635–43.

26. Koffel E, Branson M, Amundson E, et al. "Sign me up, I'm ready!": Helping patients prescribed sleeping medication engage with cognitive behavioral therapy for insomnia (CBT-I). Behav Sleep Med 2020;1–11.

27. Department of Veterans Affairs and Department of Defense. Clinical practice guideline for the management of posttraumatic stress disorder and acute stress disorder; Pocket Card. 2018. Washington, DC. Available at: https://www.healthquality.va.gov/guidelines/MH/ptsd/VADoDPTSDCPGPocketCardFinal508-082918b.pdf. Accessed October 15, 2020.

28. Chakravorty S, Morales K, Amedt J, et al. Cognitive behavioral therapy for insomnia in alcohol-dependent veterans: a randomized controlled pilot study. Alcohol Clin Exp Res 2019;43(6):1244–53.

29. Taylor D, Peterson A, Pruiksma K, et al. Impact of cognitive behavioral therapy for insomnia disorder on sleep and comorbid symptoms in military personnel: a randomized clinical trial. Sleep Res Soc 2018;41(6):1–11.

30. Kelly M, Robbins R, Martin J. Delivering cognitive behavioral therapy for insomnia in military personnel and veterans. Sleep Med Clin 2019;14:199–208.

31. Nicosia FM, Kaul B, Totten AM, et al. Leveraging telehealth to improve access to care: a qualitative evaluation of Veterans' experience with the VA TeleSleep program. BMC Health Serv Res 2021;21:77.

32. Mahfoud Y, Talin F, Streem D, et al. Sleep disorders in substance abusers: How common are they? Psychiatry 2009;6(9):38–42.

33. Substance Abuse and Mental Health Services Administration. National survey on drug use and health: veterans 2018. Available at: https://www.samhsa.gov/data/sites/default/files/reports/rpt23251/6_Veteran_2020_01_14_508.pdf. Acessed October 15, 2020.

34. Kuehner C. My military: a navy nurse practitioner's perspective on military culture and joining forces for veteran health. J Am Assoc Nurse Pract 2015;25:77–83.

35. National Institute on Drug Abuse. Drug facts: substance use and military life 2019. Available at: https://www.drugabuse.gov/sites/default/files/drugfacts_subabusemilitary.pdf. Accessed October 15, 2020.

36. Department of Veterans Affairs and Department of Defense. Clinical practice guideline for the management of substance use disorders. 2016. Washington, DC. Available at: https://www.healthquality.va.gov/guidelines/MH/sud/VADoDSUDCPGRevised22216.pdf. Accessed October 15, 2020.

37. Department of Veterans Affairs and Department of Defense. Clinical practice guideline for the management of substance use disorders stabilization pocket card. 2017. Washington, DC. Available at: https://www.healthquality.va.gov/guidelines/MH/sud/VADoDSUDCPGPocketCardStabilizationFinal.pdf. Accessed October 15, 2020.

38. Han B, Sherman S, Link A, et al. Comparison of the substance use brief screen (SUBS) to the AUDIT-C and ASSIST for detecting unhealthy alcohol and drug use in a population of hospitalized smokers. J Subst Abuse Treat 2017;79:67–74.

39. Miller M, Metrik J, Borsari B, et al. Longitudinal associations between sleep, intrusive thoughts, and alcohol problems among veterans. Alcohol Clin Exp Res 2019; 43(11):2438–45.

40. Schweizer C, Hoggatt K, Washington D, et al. Use of alcohol as a sleep aid, unhealthy drinking behaviors and sleeping pill use among women veterans. Sleep Health 2019;5:495–500.

41. Hoggatt K, Simpson T, Schweizer C, et al. Brief report: identifying women veterans with unhealth alcohol use using gender-tailored screening. Am J Addict 2018;27:97–100.

42. Department of Veterans Affairs and Department of Defense. Clinical practice guideline for the management of substance use disorders screening and treatment pocket card. 2017. Washington, DC. Available at: https://www.healthquality.va.gov/guidelines/MH/sud/VADoDSUDCPGPocketcardScreeningandTreatmentRevised081017.pdf. Accessed October 15, 2020.

Sleep Disorders and Mood, Anxiety, and Post-Traumatic Stress Disorders

Overview of Clinical Treatments in the Context of Sleep Disturbances

W. Chance Nicholson, PhD, MS, PMHNP-BC*,
Kate Pfeiffer, MSN, PMHNP-BC, PMHCNS-BC

KEYWORDS

- Sleep disturbances • Anxiety • PTSD • Mood disorders • Treatment

KEY POINTS

- Sleep disturbances can be both a risk factor for and exacerbate symptoms of anxiety, depression, and trauma-related stress.
- Alterations in sleep are extremely common in and may exacerbate generalized anxiety disorder, mood disorders, and post-traumatic stress disorder.
- Common psychotropic medications can contribute to or exacerbate sleep disorders
- Understanding the inter-relationships and symptom overlap in sleep and psychiatric disorders will help to optimize clinical care and patient outcomes.

Sufficient and restorative sleep is critical to our well-being; it provides a multisystem buffer against physiologic stress states, which is necessary for optimal physical and mental health. Sleep is a critical substrate for regulating the metabolic, immunologic, and cognitive-affective (eg, inhibitory control, emotions, memory consolidation) processes for present and future homeostatic functions. Unfortunately, sleep disorders are observed in 35% to 50% of the general population annually, with those living with a psychiatric disorder representing the highest prevalence rates.[1] Difficulty falling or staying asleep, poor sleep quality, within sleep interruptions (eg, nightmares), and excessive daytime sleepiness are the primary disturbances observed in mood disorders (ie, major depressive disorder [MDD] and bipolar disorder [BD]), generalized anxiety disorder (GAD), and post-traumatic stress disorder (PTSD). Sleep disturbances impose a

The authors have nothing to disclose.
Nell Hodgson Woodruff School of Nursing, Emory University, 1520 Clifton Road, Atlanta, GA 30322, USA
* Corresponding author. Nell Hodgson Woodruff School of Nursing, Office of Research, Emory University, 1520 Clifton Road, Office: 264, Atlanta, GA 30322.
E-mail address: william.c.nicholson@emory.edu

Nurs Clin N Am 56 (2021) 229–247
https://doi.org/10.1016/j.cnur.2021.02.003
0029-6465/21/© 2021 Elsevier Inc. All rights reserved.

nursing.theclinics.com

significant burden on the course of psychiatric treatment (eg, response), remission rates, and increase the severity and risk of relapse in mood, anxiety, and PTSDs.[2]

Increasing evidence suggests a complex inter-relationship between sleep and psychiatric disorder pathways, such that sleep disturbances represent interacting causative and/or resultant features of psychiatric disorder symptomatology, meaning that psychiatric disorders can precipitate sleep disruptions and sleep disturbances can precipitate psychiatric disorders. The common co-occurrence of psychiatric and primary sleep disorders such as insomnia, restless leg syndrome (RLS), obstructive sleep apnea (OSA), and circadian rhythm sleep disorders (CRSD) supports the likelihood of shared mechanisms underlying their psychopathology.[3] Sleep disruptions associated with sleep disorders include a multitude of both short- and long-term psychiatric sequelae, such as somatic problems, stress reactivity, resilience, psychosocial issues, anxiety, depression, memory problems, impulsivity, cardiometabolic dysfunctions, and low quality of life.[4] Given the bidirectional nature and co-occurrence of sleep disturbances in common psychiatric and sleep disorders, targeting sleep symptoms provides a critical avenue for optimizing clinical treatments and outcomes.

The purpose of this article is to focus on the clinical co-occurrence of common psychiatric (ie, mood, GAD, and PTSD) and sleep disturbances in the context of sleep disorders (ie, OSA, RLS, parasomnia, and CRSD) where psychiatric treatments are best characterized. To accomplish this goal, key diagnostic definitions are provided, a general overview of their inter-relationship to sleep disturbance follows, and then clinical psychopharmacologic and psychotherapeutic considerations for treating sleep disturbances and psychiatric disorders are provided.

CLINICAL DIAGNOSIS OF PSYCHIATRIC AND SLEEP DISORDERS

Sleep disturbance is defined by integrating a range of disorder classifications, clinical assessments (eg, subjective complaints; Insomnia Severity Index[5]; Pittsburgh Sleep Quality Index[6]), and objective haptic measures (electroencephalogram, polysomnography [PSG], and actigraphy). The fifth edition of the *Diagnostic and Statistical Manual of Mental Disorders* (2013) provides a taxonomic and diagnostic structure for clinicians and researchers alike to identify psychiatric and sleep disorders in adult populations, as well as their accompanying patterns of disturbed sleep.[7] Psychiatric and sleep symptomatology is significant clinically when impairment or disorder occurs in life domains (eg, social, personal, occupational) and interferes with quality of life. Using the DSM-5, the next section briefly defines the primary psychiatric and sleep disorders represented in this article (**Table 1**).

Psychiatric Disorders

Mood disorders consist of a spectrum of conditions including depression and BD (eg, hypomania, mania). MDD affects about 7.1% of adults (twice as common in women) in the United States every year, with a lifetime prevalence of about 20%, whereas BD affects about 2.8% of adults with a lifetime prevalence of 4.4%.[2] MDD is characterized by hallmark features of anhedonia and depressed mood along with dysregulations in neurobehavioral domains such as decreased concentration, pleasure, motivation, energy levels, changes in appetite or weight, poor sleep, and alterations in psychomotor activity. BD has 2 primary diagnostic arms (excluding cyclothymia). BD I is designated by classical manic symptoms of dysregulated mood (eg, elevated, expansive, irritable), psychosis (eg, grandiosity), decreased need for sleep, increases in speech patterns (rapid, pressured), goal-directed activities, and distractibility. Similarly, BD II is characterized by at least 1 major depressive and hypomanic episode (lasting approximately 4 days).

Table 1
Sleep disturbances and differentials

Sleep Disturbance	Patient Complaints	Differential Diagnosis
Sleep onset	Lying in bed Use of medications or substances to induce sleep	Primary insomnia RLS GAD Major depression Bipolar I and II disorders Antidepressants

Sleep maintenance	Frequent waking for known or
	  unidentifiable reasons
	Difficulty returning to sleep
		Major depression
		Bipolar I and II disorders,
		  especially when comorbid
		  with anxiety
		OAS
		Periodic limb movements
		Antidepressants

Early waking	Waking earlier than intended; unable to fall back to sleep	GAD Major depression

The lifetime general population prevalence of GAD is 9% (twice as common in women). GAD is defined as chronic, unfocused worry across multiple domains with clinically significant distress, functional impairment, and is often accompanied by poor concentration, muscle tension, restlessness, and fatigue, which may be the consequences of sleep loss. Notably, comorbid major depression is reported in up to 70% of GAD cases.[8]

The lifetime prevalence of adults living with PTSD is estimated to be 6.1% to 9.2%.[9] PTSD is characterized by an exposure to actual or threatened death, serious injury, or sexual violence that results in a cluster of stress-based symptomology. Hallmark symptoms include recurrent, intrusive trauma thoughts (nightmares, flashbacks, or marked physiologic reactions to traumatic reminders); avoidance of cognitive–emotional reminders or triggers of events (eg, memories, thoughts, or feelings); cognitive or mood dysregulations (eg, trauma-related amnesia, guilt, negative emotions, personal detachment); and altered arousal and reactivity (eg, irritability, sleep disturbance, hypervigilance).

Sleep Disorders

Sleep disorders are characterized by dysregulation in the sleep–wake spectrum. The sleep–wake spectrum represents a multimodal, circadian and physiologic homeostatic drive that coordinates the quantity, content, and timing of sleep cycles. Generally, sleep is evaluated relative to duration, onset latency, efficiency, and time awake after onset (ie, periods awake during the night). Sleep dysregulation can occur at any of the 3 different levels of consciousness (ie, wakefulness, REM sleep, and non-REM [NREM] sleep). Wakefulness represents a physiologic continuum of arousal-state transitions (typified by high-frequency alpha/beta waves, low-amplitude electroencephalogram activity) necessary for conscious, regulatory functions (eg, goal-directed behaviors). REM (paradoxic active-sleep) represents a high energy, catabolic state driven by the brainstem whereby wakefulness-like cortical activity (theta/gamma waves), electrical desynchronization, and dreams occur. NREM is a triarchic state with increasing delta and decreasing alpha waves. The 3 states are classified by N1 (a transition between wakefulness and sleep), N2 (characterizes a majority of sleep time), and N3 (deep or slow wave sleep). The deep sleep stage is characterized by slow and synchronized electrical activity.[10]

Insomnia is the most common sleep disorder and the most researched. The estimated prevalence of insomnia in the general population is 10%. Insomnia can be short term (<3 months with an identifiable stressor such as bereavement) or chronic. Chronic insomnia disorder is defined as experiencing difficulty falling asleep or staying asleep and/or early morning awakenings at least 3 times per week for at least 3 months. Insomnia occurs when there are adequate sleep conditions and opportunities (eg, nonimposed 8-hour time blocks). Furthermore, insomnia must be associated with excessive daytime sleepiness, irritability, fatigue, an increase in mental errors, and decreased concentration or memory retrieval.

CRSDs are disruptions in sleep and wakefulness resulting from physiologic, biochemical, and behavioral desynchronization of intrinsic circadian clock activity relative to external cycles (eg, light/d) or cues (eg, social activity). Central and peripheral clock synchronization occurs in the hypothalamic suprachiasmatic nuclei and is critical for regulating stress-inflammation, mood (eg, motivation, pleasure), and arousal. CRSDs can occur owing to unpredictable entrainment to chronobiological events, such as food consumption, nocturnal light exposure, irregular sleeping patterns, and frequent time zone changes.[11] The diagnostic criteria requires a persistent or recurrent pattern of sleep disturbance owing to alterations in the circadian rhythms and a sleep–wake schedule that results from and causes impairment in one's physical, occupational, social, and/or personal functional environment. The disruption must lead to either insomnia, excessive sleepiness, or a combination of both.

OSA is an increasingly common, chronic, sleep-related breathing disorder with a prevalence of 9% to 34% for adults (between 30 and 70 years of age) in the moderate to severe range.[12] It is characterized by periodic narrowing and obstruction of the pharyngeal airway (eg, snoring, gasping) during sleep that results in fatigue, nonrestorative sleep, excessive daytime sleepiness, and cognitive impairments. OSA severity is categorized using an apnea-hypopnea index (number of apnea and hypopnea events per hour of sleep). The OSA index parameter scores are mild (5–10), moderate (15–30), and severe (>30); and is diagnosed using PSG (typically performed in a sleep clinic) or home sleep device testing.

RLS is a common sensorimotor disorder with an estimated prevalence of 9% to 15%.[13] It is characterized by an uncomfortable sensory sensation in the extremities (eg, tingling, burning, pain) and akathisia (constant need to move legs, sometimes arms), which tend to occur during resting states (particularly in the evening and nighttime) and are relieved with motor activity. The sleep disturbances are accompanied by a motor sign referred to as periodic leg movements during sleep (PLMS). Sleep-related problems occur with delayed sleep onset and/or sleep maintenance insomnia and contributes to fatigue, daytime sleepiness, and a decreased ability to concentrate.

Parasomnias are a group of sleep disorders characterized by motor, sensory, or behavioral episodes (eg, acting out a dream) that occur at the onset of sleep, during sleep, and during the arousal stages from sleep. The diagnosis typically occurs via self-report and observations from persons living in the home, and video PSG. Although many different parasomnias, typically divided into NREM (eg, sleepwalking, sleep-related eating disorders) and REM disorders (eg, sleep paralysis), this article focuses primarily on nightmares (REM and NREM), because they often (50%–96%) accompany trauma-related disorders such as PTSD.

BACKGROUND AND SIGNIFICANCE

The clinical relationship between sleep disturbances and psychiatric disorders is not a novel one. In fact, Ford and Kamerow[14] (1989) provided one of the earliest epidemiologic studies suggesting insomnia's role as a precursor or predictor of mood disorder development. After this hallmark study, multiple insomnia studies have replicated these findings while also demonstrating similar relationships for GAD and PTSD.[15–17] Importantly, recent meta-analyses have also demonstrated that sleep disturbances observed during remission states predict the duration and severity of these psychiatric disorders.[18] Given this finding, sleep disturbances likely represent a prodromal signature and/or a transdiagnostic marker for affective and mood disorders; thus, it provides a target for both prevention and intervention in psychiatric disorder treatment.

Notably, targeting sleep disturbances in psychiatric disorders can pose unique challenges to mental health clinicians, such that psychopharmacologic agents may exacerbate the symptoms of primary sleep disorders. The primary treatment goals of a clinician are to decrease the negative effects of symptoms on the person living with a psychiatric disorder. Importantly, although medications are critical for treating the salient symptoms that characterize MDD, GAD, and PTSD, numerous studies suggest that select psychopharmacologic agents could negatively impact specific sleep parameters while also contributing to the development and/or exacerbation of certain sleep disorders.[2] For example, Doghramji and Jangro[19] (2016) found that persons diagnosed with MDD or GAD commonly experience insomnia and daytime somnolence when treated with selective serotonin reuptake inhibitors (SSRIs) and selective serotonin and norepinephrine reuptake inhibitors. Given the role of sleep disturbances in psychiatric sequelae development and severity, ongoing efforts are focused on understanding the bidirectional relationship underlying its effect on these commonly diagnosed disorders and improving treatment approaches.

PSYCHIATRIC DISORDERS' IMPACT ON SLEEP
Mood Disorders

Numerous studies have demonstrated that dysregulated sleep can precede the onset of mood disorders, increase the risk of developing a future mood disorder, and may be a strong predictor of relapse.[3] More recently, mood disorder studies have suggested REM and N3 disturbances that persist in remissive states predict relapse and poor treatment outcomes.[20] Given this finding, a sleeping pattern assessment in those with mood disorders provides useful context for treatment planning.

Insomnia or hypersomnia is reported by approximately 70% to 80% of persons experiencing MDD. Depression-related insomnia is categorized by sleep onset delays and frequent waking, especially in the early morning hours. Likewise, insomnia and hypersomnia are commonly observed in BD. Sleep disturbances occur interepisodically in BD, with most patients experiencing insomnia. A decreased need for sleep characterizes BD-mania with approximately 64% to 99% of persons experiencing a decreased need for sleep and longer sleep onset latency.[21] Importantly, associations exist between sleep deprivation and increased risk for inducing manic episodes. Furthermore, according to Ng and colleagues (2015),[22] persons at higher risk for developing BD or experiencing an episode demonstrate greater variability in sleep efficiency and decreased relative amplitude.

PSG studies demonstrate decreases in N3 sleep, slow-wave activity (ie, delta), REM latency, and an increased percentage of REM sleep and density in persons diagnosed with depression. Moreover, delays in sleep onset and longer periods of wakefulness after sleep onset have been related to more severe depressive symptoms.[23] Similar polysomnographic findings are demonstrated for BD. A recent actigraphy meta-analysis conducted by Tazawa and colleagues[24] (2018) demonstrated earlier awakenings and decreased daily activity in persons diagnosed with MDD when compared with controls. In remission or interepisodic states, De Crescenzo and colleagues[25] (2017) (n = 13 studies) found a similar sleep pattern in euthymic (supposed clinical stability) BD of decreased overall sleep time and efficiency, awakenings, and dysregulated sleep–wake cycles. Importantly, evidence suggests the presence of sleep disturbance in euthymic BD predicted an increased rate of suicide relative to those without sleep disturbances.

Dysregulated circadian timing, amplitude, or instability are observed in mood disorders. Although CRSDs are a feature of both depression and BD, circadian dysregulation (particularly, delayed sleep–wake phases) could be a more significant feature of BD. The effects of CRSD on both BD I and BD II with a younger onset age of BD and family history of suicide demonstrating the strongest associations. Takaesu[26] (2018) suggests that circadian disruptions correspond with low melatonin and could represent a marker for BD given decreased serum levels were found during all of phases of BD (euthymic, depressed, and manic).

Significantly increased rates of OSA are seen in patients with mood disorders. For example, a recent meta-analysis found OSA in approximately 36% of persons with MDD and 25% with BD.[27] Causal mechanisms contributing to frequency of OSA in mood disorders is unknown and is the focus of ongoing research, but is suggested to result from multiple factors (eg, cardiovascular disease, substance use, obesity). Notably, Gupta and Simpson[28] (2015) suggested increased associations were attributable to psychiatric medications (particularly, benzodiazepines).

Generalized Anxiety Disorder

A basic response to a perceived stressor, anxiety is highly associated with various sleep disturbances. Most individuals with anxiety disorders report difficulty with sleep initiation, maintenance, and decreased total sleep time compared with the general population. These subjective sleep concerns often precede the onset of GAD and are associated with the development of GAD over time. Notably, these subjective complaints are often remarkably similar for patients with primary insomnia in clinical settings.[29,30]

Of the anxiety disorders, GAD is characterized by chronic, excessive worry for a period of at least 6 months, across global domains of one's life. The worry is associated with feeling restless, poor concentration, muscle tension, and irritability. Resulting from poorly controlled worry and physiologic arousal, insomnia is a prominent symptom of GAD, with problems of sleep latency and maintenance in more than 50% of individuals. Likewise, insomnia prevalence estimates of up to 90% are observed for persons with anxiety disorders. This finding suggests a range of symptoms related to shared neurobiological pathways and successful treatment of anxiety should involve targeted insomnia interventions.[30,31] Associations between anxiety and sleep disturbances are fundamental to understanding arousal patterns and dysfunction observed in both conditions. The state of increased arousal may be related to delayed sleep initiation and frequent waking. Compared with other anxiety subtypes in DSM-5, insomnia may have a stronger interrelationship with GAD.

Individuals with GAD experience increased sleep latency, decreased overall sleep time, and variations in NREM sleep compared with the general populations, and that evidence for alterations in REM patterns is equivocal, and seems to vary across the lifespan.[29,32] Importantly, REM patterns do seem to differentiate GAD from MDD and could be a useful clinical marker in determining whether treatment should focus more on anxious or depressive symptoms in cases of co-occurrence.

Post-traumatic Stress Disorder

A constellation of sleep disruptions are observed in PTSD, with approximately 70% to 90% of persons experiencing a co-occurring sleep disorder.[33] Insomnia and parasomnias (particularly nightmares) are the most common disturbances. Decreased sleep efficiency, delayed onset, and increased frequency of awakenings characterize the insomnia observed in PTSD and are highly associated with intrusive thought symptomatology. Similar to GAD and mood disorders, insomnia is a significant risk factor for PTSD because it may precede and predict its development. A recent military study found persons with insomnia before being deployed had an increased likelihood of developing PTSD after deployment.[34] Recent studies also suggest that insomnia occurring in the initial stages of PTSD can become an independent diagnosis owing to it precipitating cognitive–behavioral dysregulation. Even with a positive response to treatment (defined as a decrease in overt symptoms), PTSD-related insomnia often persists and can cause a relapse in irritability, poor concentration, and dysregulated mood. Moreover, in the acute phases, insomnia also increases the risk of suicide in persons living with PTSD.[35]

PSG studies suggest REM-related pathology could be a key feature of PTSD. A recent meta-analytic review demonstrated decreased slow-wave activity, increased REM density over shorter periods, and increased N1 sleep in PTSD relative to controls. Interestingly, fragmented REM has been found acutely after trauma exposure and in chronic PTSD. These findings suggest that decreases in REM sleep could be an early marker both prodromally and after PTSD onset, thus providing a possible mediating role in the symptom course.[36] Given this finding, REM activity could provide a useful objective measure of psychopharmacologic agents effectiveness when prescribed to manage sleep disturbances.

Nightmares are hallmark features of PTSD and diagnostically unique relative to mood and anxiety disorders. Veterans living with PTSD are particularly vulnerable to increased occurrence ($\geq$5 times a week), severity, and distressing nightmare content when compared with controls and other trauma-exposed individuals.[37] Nightmares influence both sleep onset and maintenance because the fear of going to sleep may be secondary to trauma-related nightmares, and cause increased number of awakenings throughout the night. Van Liempt and colleagues[38] (2013) suggested that the awakenings were directly related to decreased sleep efficiency; likewise, studies have found decreased efficiency and increased awakenings are strongly correlated with magnitude of dream recall. Interestingly, nightmares have also been shown to increase apnea–hypopnea indices in OSA owing to fragmented arousal patterns.

A co-occurrence between PTSD and OSA has also been observed with rates of 13% to 83%, which is higher than OSA rates in the general population. Recent studies have found a positive correlation between apnea–hypopnea scores and PTSD symptoms severity.[28,39] A review by Schredl[40] found apneic episodes influenced heightened nightmare recall and increased negative emotions. Pagel and Kwiatkowski[41] (2010) found persons with higher apnea–hypopnea indices experienced reduced nightmares owing to impaired cognitive recall that occurs with chronic and severe OSA. Consistent with these findings, continuous positive air pressure treatment in persons with mild to moderate OSA decrease nightmare frequency, and continuous positive air pressure use in moderate to severe cases can cause an increase in frequency and recall.[42] The latter findings could provide an explanation as to why continuous positive air pressure compliance is low in persons living with PTSD.

PSYCHOPHARMACOLOGIC TREATMENTS OF PSYCHIATRIC DISORDERS WITH CONSIDERATIONS FOR PRIMARY SLEEP DISORDERS

Pharmacotherapy for psychiatric disorder symptomology includes a multitude of different classes such as benzodiazepines, nonbenzodiazepine/sedative hypnotics, selective histamine-1 receptor antagonists, melatonin receptor agonists, antidepressants, antipsychotics, and over-the-counter agents (**Table 2**). Notably, it is beyond the scope of this article to provide specific prescribing regimens (eg, dosing, phenotyping). Rather, a broad overview of common medications and select novel agents are provided to contextualize their impact on sleep disorders.

Antidepressants

An initial treatment with the more "activating" antidepressant agents such as fluoxetine (an SSRI), venlafaxine (a norepinephrine reuptake inhibitor), and desipramine (a tricyclic antidepressant [TCA]) have the highest rates of emergent insomnia. Specifically, increases in REM latency, suppressed REM sleep, and reduced sleep duration are observed. Furthermore, SSRI-induced (via omnipause neuronal inhibition) paradoxic eye movements during NREM sleep has been demonstrated and is likely underdiagnosed or misdiagnosed as normal REM sleep. Most antidepressants demonstrate an approximately 30% decrease in REM sleep parameters, but activating agents are the more likely culprit.[43] Some activating effects can be ameliorated by adjusting the dosing schedule (eg, decreasing dose, slower titration) or using less activating medications (eg, citalopram, vortioxetine). If dose adjustments are ineffective, more sedative-based antidepressants are often used.[44]

Sedative-based antidepressants (eg, doxepin, amitriptyline, mirtazapine, trazodone), specifically those blocking histaminergic and α-1 receptors, can rapidly improve sleep efficiency, increase slow-wave sleep, and decrease latency. Notably, sleep trade-offs also occur with these antidepressants; high rates of emergent somnolence (daytime sleepiness, oversedation) and weight gain are observed. This trade-off is particularly germane given insomnia and OSA comorbidities occur in approximately 30% of persons, and weight gain is a known risk factor for OSA.

Mirtazapine (a noradrenergic-specific serotonergic agent) is among the more common and effective sedative-based antidepressants used for insomnia (despite a paucity of studies examining its effects on primary insomnia), but is a significant contributor to weight gain and not recommended in those with OSA. One of the more notable effects of mirtazapine is its strong associations with treatment-emergent RLS, aggravated RLS, and PLMS. This effect is more pronounced if combined with activating SSRIs and norepinephrine reuptake inhibitors, given that increased serotonergic activity is robustly associated with increases in RLS occurrences.[45] Notably, the augmentation of bupropion (norepinephrine–dopamine reuptake inhibitor) has been shown to reduce these RLS effects.[46] 5HT2A antagonists (such as trazodone and nefazodone) help to initiate sleep and could decrease nightmare frequency in PTSD; furthermore, some benefits have also been observed in the context of OSA despite weight gain being a prominent side effect.[47] Notably, treatment-emergent or exacerbated RLS is also seen with 5HT2A antagonists. However, much like doxepin, a worsening of PLMS is not commonly observed.[48]

TCAs (such as doxepin and amitriptyline) have multiple uses in MDD, GAD, PTSD, and sleep disorders. However, their side effect profiles (eg, metabolic, cardiovascular, and cognitive) limit their use as first- and second-line agents for any given disorder. One exception is low-dose doxepin (<10 mg) owing to supposed selective histamine (H_1) receptor antagonism at lower doses, which minimizes the oversedating effects,

Table 2
Medication indications and sleep outcomes

Medication Class	Select Medication	Indication	Effects on Sleep and/or Psychiatric Disorders
SSRIs	Fluoxetine, sertraline, paroxetine, citalopram, escitalopram	MDD, GAD, PTSD	Emergent RLS and PLMS; risk of insomnia, daytime sedation, REM alterations
Serotonin antagonist and reuptake inhibitor	Trazodone, nefazodone	Primary/secondary insomnia; MDD	Does not affect OSA or RLS indices
Serotonin-norepinephrine reuptake inhibitor	Duloxetine, venlafaxine	MDD, GAD, PTSD	Emergent RLS and PLMS; risk of insomnia, daytime sedation, REM alterations
Noradrenergic and specific serotonergic antidepressant	Mirtazapine	MDD/PTSD/GAD-related insomnia	Increases RLS and OSA risk
Tricyclic antidepressants	Amitriptyline, doxepin	MDD, GAD	Amitriptyline could worsen RLS and PLMS Low dose doxepin best choice overall
Antipsychotics	Quetiapine, risperidone	BD I; PTSD-related sleep disturbances	Increases metabolic risk factors (eg, obesity, insulin dysregulation) that exacerbate or contribute to development of OSA, RLS
Mood stabilizers	Depakote, carbamazepine	BD I, BD II	Can increase vividness of nightmares in PTSD
Melatonin receptor agonist	Melatonin	Jet lag, shift-work disorder, circadian rhythm disorders	Could help reduce the metabolic side effects from antipsychotics; Could provide circadian regulatory benefits in BD
Benzodiazepines; nonbenzodiazepines sedative hypnotics	Clonazepam, alprazolam, temazepam; zolpidem; eszopiclone	Short-term insomnia; acute mania, GAD, mixed anxiety-depression	NREM and REM parasomnias (caution in PTSD)
Nonbenzodiazepine/sedative-hypnotics	Zolpidem, eszopiclone	Primary, transient, chronic insomnia; insomnia related to MDD/GAD/PTSD	Possible use in PTSD and OSA
Alpha-blockers	Prazosin	PTSD-related nightmares	Possibly increases risk of OSA

impaired memory consolidation, and cognitive impairments observed in other antihistamines (eg, diphenhydramine) and TCAs.[49] Notably, higher doses of doxepin retain similar side effects as those observed in other TCAs owing to increased norepinephrine, serotonergic, and anticholinergic activity.

A recent meta-analysis found low-dose doxepin increased sleep maintenance, decreased the number of awakenings, and increased sleep efficiency and duration. Improvements in OSA apneic–hypopnea episodes are also reported. Conversely, although amitriptyline is commonly used for sleep disturbances, a recent Cochrane Review did not support its use in insomnia. Similar to doxepin, lower doses have been shown to improve subjective sleep quality; however, unlike doxepin, RLS aggravation and the side effect profile remains a concern. On balance, low-dose doxepin seems to be the most effective agent with the lowest risk of exacerbating sleep disorders.[50]

Mood Stabilizers and Antipsychotics

Medications used to treat bipolar-associated depression and mania are often referred to as general mood stabilizers. Mood stabilizers include atypical antipsychotics, lithium, and anticonvulsants. All of the general mood stabilizers precipitate sleep to varying degrees, but also tend to promote daytime sedation. These sleep-promoting qualities have resulted in their being used off-label to treat insomnia.

Valproate has been shown to decrease sleep onset time, improve sleep efficiency (particularly in N1 and N3), and decrease PLMS during arousal phases. Similarly, although research is lacking, lamotrigine and carbamazepine demonstrate some efficacy in RLS by decreasing its overall severity and also tend to cause less weight gain than valproate. To date, studies do not demonstrate any efficacy in insomnia.[51] Some evidence suggests an effect of lithium on CRSD; modifications to circadian rhythms and their associated clock genes have been observed. These modifications are augmented when paired with sleep deprivation therapy.[52] Importantly, in the absence of a mood disorder diagnosis, research is lacking to support lithium's use in CRSDs, nor does it seem to have any effect on other sleep disorders.

Antipsychotics (eg, quetiapine and risperidone) have also demonstrated some improvement in subjective sleep quality (owing to rapid onset), decreased awakenings, increased sleep duration, increased N3 sleep, and decreased REM movements. However, much like anticonvulsants, rigorous studies are lacking that support their use in insomnia. Anecdotally, benefits are observed in a subset of persons experiencing sleep disturbances (particularly PTSD).[53] Notably, most antipsychotics have been shown to exacerbate or cause RLS.[54] Antipsychotics have also been explored as potential agents for nightmares with low-dose risperidone and quetiapine demonstrating some effect on reducing frequency.[55] Conversely, anticonvulsant agents (particularly valproate) can increase vividness of dreams. Although it is unclear whether or not mood stabilizers cause or promote nightmares, it does seem that they can increase the intensity and dream recall potential of trauma-related nightmares.

Importantly, the metabolic side effects of these medications are particularly relevant in the context of precipitating or exacerbating OSA. Interestingly, according to a recent meta-analysis, melatonin receptor agonists have demonstrated the ability to decrease or even eliminate the metabolic side effects of atypical antipsychotics.[56] Melatonin is one of the most common over-the-counter medications used for sleep disturbances. Its effectiveness in insomnia is mixed; however, multiple studies support its use in jet lag, RLS, and select CRSDs.[57] Given that many individuals with mood disorders have CRSDs, the use of melatonin to address the metabolic problems associated with atypical antipsychotics seems particularly germane.

Benzodiazepines and Nonbenzodiazepine Hypnotics

Benzodiazepines (eg, clonazepam, temazepam) are often prescribed for GAD and insomnia related to anxiety or stress owing to subjective increases in sleep efficiency, maintenance, and rapid sleep induction. Although originally designed for short-term use, they have increasingly been used for the longer term management of chronic anxiety and other sleep disturbances (particularly primary NREM and REM parasomnias). Their efficacy in parasomnias has led to an increased use in PTSD-related nightmares and insomnia, although their use is discouraged given risk of tolerance, dependency, and concerns they negatively impact PTSD neural pathways and ongoing treatments (eg, psychotherapy). Because benzodiazepines affect gamma aminobutyric acid, they are also commonly used adjunctively in RLS and PLMS to target arousal indices. Importantly, randomized controlled trials are lacking to support their use as a primary treatment for RLS.[58] Another concern is the high comorbidity rates between PTSD and OSA given benzodiazepines can exacerbate apneic episodes owing to their central nervous system depressing properties.

In cases of PTSD and OSA comorbidities, clinicians often prescribe nonbenzodiazepines (eg, zolpidem, eszopiclone). A recent meta-analysis supports this practice because they exert milder central nervous system effects, increase sleep quality and efficiency, and have little effect on sleep apnea.[59] However, the risks of dependency and tolerance are a concern for these medications as well. In general, nonbenzodiazepines are not recommended for mood disorders and GAD sleep disturbances given their inability to improve anxiety or depressive symptoms and to increase the risk for suicide.[60] In addition to their addictive potential, the most problematic side effect of both benzodiazepines and nonbenzodiazepines is their potential to induce somnambulism (particularly zolpidem), because this factor puts persons in high-risk situations while in a sleeping state (eg, driving a car).[61] In general, these medications should be avoided unless other interventions have failed and the risk–benefit has been considered.

Other Medications

Selective histamine-1 receptor antagonists such as hydroxyzine are used for insomnia, anxiety, and PTSD-related nightmares. A recent PTSD study found that hydroxyzine decreased nightmares and improved overall sleep when compared with a placebo, but other studies have failed to replicate these findings. Differently than diphenhydramine, hydroxyzine does not seem to exacerbate PLMS and RLS.[62] The alpha-blocker prazosin is considered the gold standard for treating nightmares; it is the only medication that demonstrates efficacy, although a research has also challenged its overall effectiveness. Prazosin increases REM percentages and period duration, while increasing total sleep time. Its effect on REM activity is suggested to underlie its ability to decrease nightmares. A similar medication, doxazosin, is also being studied for PTSD nightmares.[63]

Cannabinoids (eg, nabilone and dronabinol) are suggested to have potential short-term benefits in sleep apnea (specifically in serotonin-implicated apneas). Furthermore, emerging evidence has suggested their potential use in nightmare reduction, REM dysregulation, and excessive daytime sleepiness,[64] all of which have implications for mood disorders, GAD, and PTSD. Importantly, the long-term effects are more equivocal; studies have found decreased sleep latency induced by cannabinoids might decrease the overall quality of sleep. Additionally, recent research has also suggested differing responses to cannabinoids (likely owing to receptor-level activity) in the context of nightmares such that increases in frequency have been observed.

Ketamine, a novel and rapid-acting antidepressant, was recently approved for MDD with suicidality given its ability to decrease overt depressive symptoms within a 24-hour period. Recent studies have also explored its use in CRSDs, given the desynchronization occurs in a subset of persons diagnosed with MDD, and is correlated to symptom severity. The findings suggested that ketamine could potentially modulate clock genes to influence circadian timing, which is a primary driver of CRSD pathology; furthermore, increases in REM sleep and neurotrophic factors (brain-derived neurotrophic factors) have also been observed.[65,66]

For optimal sleep-promoting benefits, medication therapies should generally be focused on early initiation, low dosing, regimented administration (eg, best timing for sleep onset), and as a part of a more holistic intervention protocol, including nonpharmacologic therapy, to improve sleep-promoting behaviors (eg, decreased stimulation, light therapy). Options should consider maximizing therapeutic benefits to target overlapping symptomatology and decrease polypharmacy whenever feasible. When pharmacotherapy is used to target sleep disturbance and/or comorbid sleep disorders, various factors should be considered:

- Symptom pattern of sleep disturbance
- Comorbid conditions and contraindications
- Past treatment response
- Patient's own perceptions, preferences, and treatment goals.

BEHAVIORAL AND CHRONOMODULATION THERAPIES

Although pharmacologic treatments provide immediate relief, they are often insufficient to address long-term dysfunctional sleep behaviors and distorted thoughts about sleep. Over time, individual thoughts, actions, and affects around sleep contribute to poor sleep habits that exacerbate distorted beliefs and expectations. These symptoms may present as irregular bedtime behaviors, spending too much time in bed, or sleep avoidant behaviors.

Coupled with improving sleep hygiene behaviors (eg, routine) and directed at improving associations between going to bed and falling asleep, cognitive behavioral therapy for insomnia (CBT-I), is currently considered a first-choice treatment for long-term dysfunctional sleep disturbances such as psychophysiological arousal and chronic insomnia. CBT-I integrates well-validated cognitive therapy commonly used in the treatment of mood disorders and hyperarousal with psychoeducation and behavioral strategies, such as sleep hygiene, relaxation training, stimulus control therapy, sleep restriction therapy, and cognitive therapy. Although CBT-I is provided via specialty-trained psychotherapists, elements of CBT-I can be implemented in various medical settings using various cognitive and behavioral strategies (**Table 3**). It is safe and effective, with superior long-term effects compared with sleep medication, and lasting benefits without rebound insomnia frequently seen in cessation of medications.[67,68] Although CBT-I does not directly target worry, anxiety, or mood symptoms, it has shown efficacy in decreasing the subjective complaints of insomnia, depression severity, and increasing the overall quality of sleep in depression and GAD.[69] CBT-I can be initiated concurrently with hypnotic medication or as it is being tapered. Despite its effectiveness, clinicians should consider issues around the cost and compliance of CBT-I.

Sleep disturbances in PTSD, particularly nightmares, are among the most difficult to treat owing to modest responses to pharmacotherapy. Imagery rehearsal therapy is an emerging behavioral intervention that has demonstrated the ability to reduce PTSD-related sleep disturbances (nightmares and insomnia) and general trauma symptoms.

Table 3
Sleep-related behavioral interventions

Behavioral Method	Description	Techniques
CBT-I	Used to identify and change maladaptive, or unhelpful, thoughts, beliefs, and behaviors related to sleep.	Challenge unhelpful beliefs about sleep Thought records to address rumination
Progressive muscle relaxation	Decreases stimulation, arousal, and rumination when trying to relax in preparation for sleep	Guided imagery Paced breathing activities Focused tension and relaxation of major muscle groups
Stimulus control	Helps patients to identify and manage frustrating associations between sleep, bedtime routines, and insomnia and strengthens bed and bedroom as sleep cues	Go to bed only when sleepy Keep bedroom dark and quiet Set a routine sleep schedule Do not nap Use bed for sleep only (no work, worry, or planning in bed)
Sleep restriction/activity scheduling	Structured activity scheduling designed to limit time spent in bed designated only for sleeping	Avoid napping Maintain fixed wake time and adjust bedtime based on sleep efficiency
Sleep hygiene promotion	Identify and decrease modifiable lifestyle behaviors that perpetuate insomnia and enhance sleep promoting activities	Avoid stimulants Limit alcohol Timing exercise and screen time away from bedtime Creation of a comfortable sleep environment.

Unfortunately, at present, recent meta-analyses demonstrate similar improvement in nightmare frequency, PTSD symptoms, and overall sleep quality when comparing imagery rehearsal therapy and prazosin.[70] Given this caveat, novel approaches are still critically needed to address PTSD-related sleep disturbances. Photobiomodulation (eg, light therapy) could provide one such approach as a recent study by Naeser and colleagues[71] demonstrated improvements in sleep quality, cognitive performance, and decreased PTSD symptoms after applying red and near infrared light.

Photoreceptors, containing photopigment melanopsin, with sensitivity to blue wavelength lights were recently discovered in the retinal ganglion. This discovery has allowed for novel innovations in photobiomodulation to modulate biological clocks, which have also recently been applied to mood disorders.[72] For example, using clinically calibrated bright lighting throughout the day (eg, 10,000 lux in the morning and 7000 midday), studies have shown a decrease in manic episodes and a decreased severity of depressive states; furthermore, improvements in subjective and total sleep quality were also observed. Emerging research also supports light therapy during the remissive states as a mechanism for decreasing mood disorder relapse. Light therapy during remission has been shown to regulate sleep homeostasis be decreasing insomnia, increasing sleep length, and stabilizing circadian rhythms (eg, sleep phase delay) via melanopsin induction.[73] Recent light therapy studies have shown its ability to modulate delta sleep activity along with exerting an antidepressant effect, which suggests an increased role for light therapy in precision medicine. Other noninvasive, neuromodulatory therapies commonly used in mood, anxiety, and PTSDs have also recently demonstrated their effect on sleep disturbances.

In the context of sleep disturbance, noninvasive neuromodulation (eg, repetitive transcranial magnetic stimulation and transcranial direct current stimulation) has primarily focused on inhibiting protocols that aim to decrease hyperarousal states during the course of sleep.[74] For example, the induced magnetic field of repetitive transcranial magnetic stimulation modulates cortical excitability and elicits specific slow wave and sleep spindle oscillations, which regulates motor and circadian activity. A recent study demonstrated (repetitive transcranial magnetic stimulation) improves sleep quality in insomnia, episodic decreased in RLS, and airflow in OSA (decreasing apneic episodes).[75] Transcranial direct current stimulation has also been shown to improve sleep disorder parameters via modulating cortical activity. Jung and Jun[76] (2018) found improvements in chronic insomnia (eg, total sleep time, latency, and efficiency) after 1 month of transcranial direct current stimulation. Another such neuromodulatory therapy is auditory stimulation. Auditory stimulation induces single, slow oscillations (or K-complexes) that entrains sleep wave activity for increased memory consolidation and improvement in sleep disorder parameters.[77] Notably, given neuromodulation is a novel approach to treating sleep disturbances, recommendations for optimal stimulation protocols are lacking.

SUMMARY

This article examined the impacts and implications of psychiatric disorders and sleep disturbances in the context of sleep disorders. Sleep disturbances represent a prodromal signature and/or a transdiagnostic marker for affective and mood disorders. Despite a high comorbidity between psychiatric and sleep disorders, sleep disturbances are often viewed as secondary or consequential to PTSD, GAD, and mood disorder pathology. As a result, sleep disorders can go undiagnosed years after onset, which could lead to increased relapses in psychiatric symptoms, increased severity, precipitation of acute episodes, and contribute to chronicity.

Compounding this lack of recognition and augmenting negative outcomes is the effect psychotropic treatments can have on the development or exacerbation of RLS, PLMS, insomnia, parasomnias, OSA, and CRSD. The early recognition of sleep disturbances, even before being diagnosed with a psychiatric disorder, could drastically improve the course and impact of these conditions via early intervention with carefully selected psychopharmacologic agents and/or neurobehavioral therapies. Furthermore, mental health collaborations with sleep clinics and/or neurology could provide more objective diagnostics (eg, PSG, electroencephalogram) and precision in prescribing regimens to reduce symptom exacerbation and assist earlier identification.

CLINICS CARE POINTS

- Assess patients with psychiatric disorders and sleep difficulties for insomnia and related sleep disorders
- Although the symptoms and treatments overlap, primary sleep disorders should be identified and treated as such in the context of psychiatric disorders.
- When optimizing pharmacotherapy, consider the impact of intended and side effects on independent and/or interrelated sleep disorders.

- Cognitive therapy approaches for insomnia overlap with best practices for GAD and depression, and may be preferred over sedative hypnotic pharmacologic monotherapy for chronic symptoms.
- Consider pharmacologic management that can target sleep disturbance and affective symptoms simultaneously, decreasing polypharmacy.
- Most medications for mood and anxiety disorders will impact sleep.
- Sleep disorders both increase the risk for the development of mental disorders, contribute to severity, and worsen psychiatric outcomes, which positions sleep as a priority clinical target.
- All patients with sleep disturbance or comorbid sleep disorder should adhere to good sleep hygiene.

REFERENCES

1. ter Heege FM, Mijnster T, van Veen MM, et al. The clinical relevance of early identification and treatment of sleep disorders in mental health care: protocol of a randomized control trial. BMC Psychiatry 2020;20(1):331.
2. Hombali A, Seow E, Yuan Q, et al. Prevalence and correlates of sleep disorder symptoms in psychiatric disorders. Psychiatry Res 2019;279:116–22.
3. Fang H, Tu S, Sheng J, et al. Depression in sleep disturbance: a review on a bidirectional relationship, mechanisms and treatment. J Cell Mol Med 2019;23(4):2324–32.
4. Medic G, Wille M, Hemels M. Short- and long-term health consequences of sleep disruption. Nat Sci Sleep 2017;9:151–61.
5. Bastien C. Validation of the Insomnia Severity Index as an outcome measure for insomnia research. Sleep Med 2001;2(4):297–307.
6. Buysse DJ, Reynolds CF, Monk TH, et al. The Pittsburgh sleep quality index: a new instrument for psychiatric practice and research. Psychiatry Res 1989; 28(2):193–213.
7. Association AP. Diagnostic and statistical manual of mental disorders. 5th edition. Washington: American Psychiatric Publishing; 2013 (DSM-5).
8. Kessler RC, DuPont RL, Berglund P, et al. Impairment in pure and comorbid generalized anxiety disorder and major depression at 12 months in two national surveys. Am J Psychiatry 1999;156(12):1915–23.
9. Koenen K, Ratanatharathorn A, Ng L, et al. Posttraumatic stress disorder in the World Mental Health Surveys. Psychol Med 2017;47(13):2260–74.
10. Pavlova K, Latreille V. Sleep disorders. Am J Med 2019;132(3):292–9.
11. Carmassi C, Palagini L, Caruso D, et al. Systematic review of sleep disturbances and circadian sleep desynchronization in autism spectrum disorder: toward an integrative model of a self-reinforcing loop. Front Psychiatry 2019;10:336.
12. Garvey JF, Pengo MF, Drakatos P, et al. Epidemiological aspects of obstructive sleep apnea. J Thorac Dis 2015;7(5):920–9.
13. Ruppert E. Restless arms syndrome: prevalence, impact, and management strategies. Neuropsychiatr Dis Treat 2019;15:1737–50.
14. Ford DE, Kamerow DB. Epidemiologic study of sleep disturbances and psychiatric disorders. An opportunity for prevention? JAMA 1989;262:1479–84.
15. Harvey AG. Sleep and circadian functioning: critical mechanisms in the mood disorders? Annu Rev Clin Psychol 2011;7:297–319.
16. Chung KH, Li CY, Kuo SY, et al. Risk of psychiatric disorders in patients with chronic insomnia and sedative-hypnotic prescription: a nationwide population-based follow-up study. J Clin Sleep Med 2015;11:543–51.

17. Wang HE, Campbell-Sills L, Kessler RC, et al. Predeployment insomnia is associated with post-deployment post-traumatic stress disorder and suicidal ideation in US Army soldiers. Sleep 2019;42:zsy229.
18. Richards A, Kanady JC, Neylan TC. Sleep disturbance in PTSD and other anxiety-related disorders: an updated review of clinical features, physiological characteristics, and psychological and neurobiological mechanisms. Neuropsychopharmacology 2020;45:55–73.
19. Doghramji K, Jangro WC. Adverse effects of psychotropic medications on sleep. Psychiatr Clin North Am 2016;39(3):487–502.
20. Rumble ME, White KH, Benca RM. Sleep disturbances in mood disorders. Psychiatr Clin North Am 2015;38(4):743–59.
21. Steardo L, de Filippis R, Carbone EA, et al. Sleep disturbance in bipolar disorder: neuroglia and circadian rhythms. Front Psychiatry 2019;10:501.
22. Ng TH, Chung K-F, Ho FY-Y, et al. Sleep-wake disturbance in interepisode bipolar disorder and high-risk individuals: a systematic review and meta-analysis. Sleep Med Rev 2015;20:46–58.
23. Luik AI, Zuurbier LA, Direk N, et al. 24-hour activity rhythm and sleep disturbances in depression and anxiety: a population-based study of middle-aged and older persons. Depress Anxiety 2015;32(9):684–92.
24. Tazawa Y, Wada M, Mitsukura Y, et al. Actigraphy for evaluation of mood disorders: a systematic review and meta-analysis. J Affect Disord 2019;253:257–69.
25. De Crescenzo F, Economou A, Sharpley AL, et al. Actigraphic features of bipolar disorder: a systematic review and meta-analysis. Sleep Med Rev 2017;33:58–69.
26. Takaesu Y. Circadian rhythm in bipolar disorder: a review of the literature. Psychiatry Clin Neurosci 2018;72(9):673–82.
27. Stubbs B, Vancampfort D, Veronese N, et al. The prevalence and predictors of obstructive sleep apnea in major depressive disorder, bipolar disorder and schizophrenia: a systematic review and meta-analysis. J Affect Disord 2016; 197:259–67.
28. Gupta MA, Simpson FC. Obstructive sleep apnea and psychiatric disorders: a systematic review. J Clin Sleep Med 2015;11:165–75.
29. Cox RC, Olatunji BO. A systematic review of sleep disturbance in anxiety and related disorders. J Anxiety Disord 2016;37:104–29.
30. Uhde TW, Cortese BM, Vedeniapin A. Anxiety and sleep problems: emerging concepts and theoretical treatment implications. Curr Psychiatry Rep 2009; 11(4):269–76.
31. Johnson EO, Roth T, Breslau N. The association of insomnia with anxiety disorders and depression: exploration of the direction of risk. J Psychiatr Res 2006; 40(8):700–8.
32. Papadimitriou GN, Linkowski P. Sleep disturbance in anxiety disorders. Int Rev Psychiatry Abingdon Engl 2005;17(4):229–36.
33. Lewis C, Lewis K, Kitchiner N, et al. Sleep disturbance in post-traumatic stress disorder (PTSD): a systematic review and meta-analysis of actigraphy studies. Eur J Psychotraumatol 2020;11(1):1767349.
34. Gehrman P, Seelig AD, Jacobson IG, et al. Predeployment sleep duration and insomnia symptoms as risk factors for new-onset mental health disorders following military deployment. Sleep 2013;36(7):1009–18.
35. Cox RC, Taylor S, Strachan E, et al. Insomnia and posttraumatic stress symptoms: evidence of shared etiology. Psychiatry Res 2020;286:112548.
36. de Boer M, Nijdam MJ, Jongedijk RA, et al. The spectral fingerprint of sleep problems in post-traumatic stress disorder. Sleep 2020;43(4):zsz269.

37. de Dassel T, Wittmann L, Protic S, et al. Association of posttraumatic nightmares and psychopathology in a military sample. Psychol Trauma Theor Res Pract Policy 2018;10(4):475–81.
38. van Liempt S, van Zuiden M, Westenberg H, et al. Impact of impaired sleep on the development of PTSD symptoms in combat veterans: a prospective longitudinal cohort study. Depress Anxiety 2013;30(5):469–74.
39. Zhang Y, Weed JG, Ren R, et al. Prevalence of obstructive sleep apnea in patients with posttraumatic stress disorder and its impact on adherence to continuous positive airway pressure therapy: a meta-analysis. Sleep Med 2017;36:125–32.
40. Schredl M. Dreams in patients with sleep disorders. Sleep medicine reviews 2009;13(3):215–21.
41. Pagel JF, Kwiatkowski C. The nightmares of sleep apnea: nightmare frequency declines with increasing apnea hypopnea index. J Clin Sleep Med 2010;6(1):69–73.
42. Pagel JF. Sleep apnea and PTSD. Post-traumatic stress disorder. Cham: Springer; 2020. p. 125–31. https://doi.org/10.1007/978-3-030-55909-0_15.
43. Horne J. REM sleep vs exploratory wakefulness: alternatives within adult 'sleep debt'? Sleep Med Rev 2019;50:101252.
44. Wichniak A, Wierzbicka A, Wałęcka M, et al. Effects of Antidepressants on sleep. Curr Psychiatry Rep 2017;19(9):63.
45. Rissardo J, Caprara AF. Mirtazapine-associated movement disorders: a literature review. Tzu Chi Med J 2020;32(4):318.
46. Rao N. The overlap between sleep disorders and psychiatric disorders. In: Sedky K, Nazir R, Bennett D, editors. Sleep Medicine and Mental Health. Cham: Springer; 2020. p. 343–73. https://doi.org/10.1007/978-3-030-44447-1_17.
47. Gaisl T, Haile SR, Thiel S, et al. Efficacy of pharmacotherapy for OSA in adults: a systematic review and network meta-analysis. Sleep Med Rev 2019;46:74–86.
48. Kolla BP, Mansukhani MP, Bostwick JM. The influence of antidepressants on restless legs syndrome and periodic limb movements: a systematic review. Sleep Med Rev 2018;38:131–40.
49. Reynolds AC, Adams RJ. Treatment of sleep disturbance in older adults. J Pharm Pract Res 2019;49(3):296–304.
50. Yeung W-F, Chung K-F, Yung K-P, et al. Doxepin for insomnia: a systematic review of randomized placebo-controlled trials. Sleep Med Rev 2015;19:75–83.
51. Oldham MA, Lee HB. Mental health disorders associated with RLS. In: Manconi M, García-Borreguero D, editors. Restless Legs Syndrome/Willis Ekbom Disease. New York: Springer; 2017. p. 21–43. https://doi.org/10.1007/978-1-4939-6777-3_2.
52. Wirz-Justice A, Benedetti F. Perspectives in affective disorders: clocks and sleep. Eur J Neurosci 2019;51(1):346–65.
53. Thompson W, Quay TAW, Rojas-Fernandez C, et al. Atypical antipsychotics for insomnia: a systematic review. Sleep Med 2016;22:13–7.
54. Aggarwal S, Dodd S, Berk M. Restless leg syndrome associated with atypical antipsychotics: current status, pathophysiology, and clinical implications. Curr Drug Saf 2015;10(2):98–105.
55. Morgenthaler TI, Auerbach S, Casey KR, et al. Position paper for the treatment of nightmare disorder in adults: an American Academy of Sleep Medicine position paper. J Clin Sleep Med 2018;14(6):1041–55.

56. Igwe SC, Brigo F. Does melatonin and melatonin agonists improve the metabolic side effects of atypical antipsychotics?: a systematic review and meta-analysis of randomized controlled trials. Clin Psychopharmacol Neurosci 2018;16(3):235–45.

57. Williams WPT, McLin DE, Dressman MA, et al. Comparative review of approved melatonin agonists for the treatment of circadian rhythm sleep-wake disorders. Pharmacother J Hum Pharmacol Drug Ther 2016;36(9):1028–41.

58. Carlos K, Prado GF, Teixeira CD, et al. Benzodiazepines for restless legs syndrome. Cochrane Database Syst Rev 2017;3(3):CD006939.

59. Zhang XJ, Li QY, Wang Y, et al. The effect of non-benzodiazepine hypnotics on sleep quality and severity in patients with OSA: a meta-analysis. Sleep Breath 2014;18(4):781–9.

60. Sateia MJ, Buysse DJ, Krystal AD, et al. Clinical practice guideline for the pharmacologic treatment of chronic insomnia in adults: an American Academy of Sleep Medicine clinical practice guideline. J Clin Sleep Med 2017;13(02):307–49.

61. Royant-Parola S, Kovess V, Brion A, et al. Do hypnotics increase the risk of driving accidents or near miss accidents due to hypovigilance? The effects of sex, chronic sleepiness, sleep habits and sleep pathology. PLoS One 2020;15(7): e0236404.

62. Di Fabio R, Casali C, Vadalà R, et al. Hydroxyzine hydrochloride in familial restless legs syndrome. Can J Neurol Sci 2010;37(3):406–7.

63. El-Solh AA. Management of nightmares in patients with posttraumatic stress disorder: current perspectives. Nat Sci Sleep 2018;10:409–20.

64. Babson KA, Sottile J, Morabito D. Cannabis, cannabinoids, and sleep: a review of the literature. Curr Psychiatry Rep 2017;19(4):23.

65. Orozco-Solis R, Montellier E, Aguilar-Arnal L, et al. A circadian genomic signature common to ketamine and sleep deprivation in the anterior cingulate cortex. Biol Psychiatry 2017;82(5):351–60.

66. Duncan WC, Slonena E, Hejazi NS, et al. Motor-activity markers of circadian timekeeping are related to ketamine's rapid antidepressant properties. Biol Psychiatry 2017;82(5):361–9.

67. Murawski B, Wade L, Plotnikoff RC, et al. A systematic review and meta-analysis of cognitive and behavioral interventions to improve sleep health in adults without sleep disorders. Sleep Med Rev 2018;40:160–9.

68. Sweetman A, Lack L, McEvoy RD, et al. Cognitive behavioural therapy for insomnia reduces sleep apnoea severity: a randomised controlled trial. ERJ Open Res 2020;6(2):00161–2020.

69. Trauer JM, Qian MY, Doyle JS, et al. Cognitive behavioral therapy for chronic insomnia: a systematic review and meta-analysis. Ann Intern Med 2015;163(3): 191–204.

70. Yücel DE, van Emmerik AAP, Souama C, et al. Comparative efficacy of imagery rehearsal therapy and prazosin in the treatment of trauma-related nightmares in adults: a meta-analysis of randomized controlled trials. Sleep Med Rev 2020; 50:101248.

71. Naeser MA, Zafonte R, Krengel MH, et al. Significant improvements in cognitive performance post-transcranial, red/near-infrared light-emitting diode treatments in chronic, mild traumatic brain injury: open-protocol study. J Neurotrauma 2014;31(11):1008–17.

72. Benedetti F. Rate of switch from bipolar depression into mania after morning light therapy: a historical review. Psychiatry Res 2018;261:351–6.

73. Maruani J, Geoffroy PA. Bright light as a personalized precision treatment of mood disorders. Front Psychiatry 2019;10:85.

74. Herrero Babiloni A, Bellemare A, Beetz G, et al. The effects of non-invasive brain stimulation on sleep disturbances among different neurological and neuropsychiatric conditions: a systematic review. Sleep Med Rev 2021;55:101381.
75. Nardone R, Sebastianelli L, Versace V, et al. Effects of repetitive transcranial magnetic stimulation in subjects with sleep disorders. Sleep Med 2020;71:113–21.
76. Jung K, Jun J. Efficacy of transcranial direct-current stimulation on chronic insomnia. Brain Stimulation 2019;12(2):557.
77. Geiser T, Hertenstein E, Fehér K, et al. Targeting arousal and sleep through noninvasive brain stimulation to improve mental health. Neuropsychobiology 2020; 79(4–5):284–92.

Sleep and Neurological Disorders

Sleep in Persons Living with Alzheimer's Disease and Related Dementias

María de los Ángeles Ordóñez, DNP, APRN, GNP-BC, PMHNP-BC, CDP, FAANP, FAAN[a,b,c,]*, Patricia de los Ángeles Ordóñez, MS, CDP[d,e,f,g]

KEYWORDS

- Sleep disorders • Older adults • Alzheimer's disease and related dementias
- Behavioral and psychological symptoms of dementia

KEY POINTS

- Aging is associated with several well-documented changes in sleep and in the sleep-wake cycle.
- Sleep-wake cycle disturbances are common in dementia of Alzheimer's disease and Lewy bodies.
- Sleep disturbances in persons living with Alzheimer's disease and related dementias can negatively affect the health of the caregivers.
- Nonpharmacologic approaches, including psychological, behavioral, and environmental interventions, should be strongly considered as first-line treatment of persons living with Alzheimer's disease and related dementias who experience sleep disorders.

OVERVIEW OF SLEEP DISORDERS

In 2017, more than 50 million Americans were diagnosed with chronic sleep disorders.[1] Current evidence supports the finding that 50 million to 70 million people in the US have 1 or several sleep disorders. "A general consensus has developed from population-based studies that approximately 30% of a variety of adult samples drawn from different countries report one or more of the symptoms of insomnia: difficulty initiating sleep, difficulty maintaining sleep, waking up too early, and in some

[a] Louis and Anne Green Memory and Wellness Center of the Christine E. Lynn College of Nursing (CELCON), Florida Atlantic University (FAU), FAU CELCON; [b] Alzheimer's Disease Initiative, Florida Department of Elder Affairs; [c] Federal Advisory Council on Alzheimer's Research, Care, and Services, US Department of Health and Human Services, 777 Glades Rd, Bldg. AZ-79, Boca Raton, FL 33431, USA; [d] Nova Southeastern University (NSU), College of Psychology; [e] Care, Supportive Services, and Outreach Coordinator, Louis and Anne Green Memory; [f] Wellness Center of the Christine E. Lynn College of Nursing (CELCON), Florida Atlantic University (FAU); [g] Alzheimer's Disease Initiative, Florida Department of Elder Affairs, 777 Glades Rd, Bldg. AZ-79, Boca Raton, FL 33431, USA
* Corresponding author.
E-mail address: Mordone3@health.fau.edu

Nurs Clin N Am 56 (2021) 249–263
https://doi.org/10.1016/j.cnur.2021.02.004
0029-6465/21/Published by Elsevier Inc.

cases, nonrestorative or poor quality of sleep."[2] Based on data collected and analyzed by Statista[3] in 2019, only 32% of adults aged 30 to 59 years and 46% of adults aged 60 years and older reported not having any sleeping problems; 35% of adults and 48% of older adults reported having trouble staying asleep throughout the night.

The American Psychiatric Association refers to the Diagnostic and Statistical Manual of Mental Disorders (DSM) to classify, diagnose, and describe mental disorders. The DSM has undergone revisions since its initial publication; this article refers to the DSM in its current fifth edition (DSM-5).

Sleep disorders are classified within the DSM-5 as disorders that result in daytime distress and impairment; individuals with sleep-wake disorders typically present self-reported "dissatisfaction regarding the quality, timing, and amount of sleep they obtain."[4] In the DSM-5, 10 sleep-wake disorders or disorder groups are included; these are insomnia, hypersomnolence, narcolepsy, breathing-related disorders (such as obstructive sleep apnea [OSA]), circadian rhythm sleep-wake disorders, non–rapid eye movement (NREM) sleep arousal disorders, nightmare disorder, rapid eye movement (REM) sleep behavior disorder, restless legs syndrome, and substance/medication-induced sleep disorder. **Fig. 1** lists the primary sleep-wake disorders among the general population.[4]

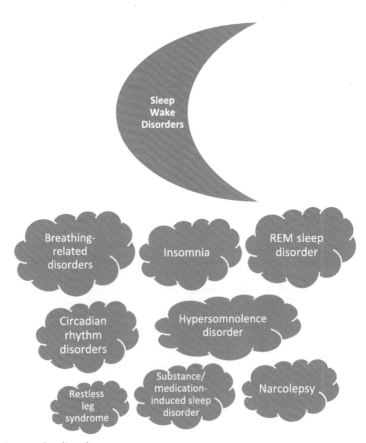

Fig. 1. Sleep-wake disorders.

There is an overlap of symptoms between sleep-wake disorders and comorbidities with other psychological and psychiatric conditions, namely depression, bipolar disorder, and schizophrenia. Sleep-wake disorders may be related directly to the pathophysiology of psychiatric illness or may come about as a reactionary response to different modalities implemented to treat a psychiatric illness or another psychological disorder. Antipsychotics have been shown to produce weight gain, leading to obstructive sleep apnea, and opioid use may produce central sleep apnea and restless leg syndrome, all of which have been shown to negatively affect quality of sleep.[5]

Evidence supports a link between psychopharmacologic intervention implementation and use, narcotic use and abuse, and the prevalence and symptoms of sleep-wake disorders; "antidepressants are known to induce a number of sleep disorders including NREM parasomnias (sleep talking, sleep walking) as well as REM parasomnias (REM sleep behavior disorder) and restless legs syndrome."[4] Opioid use has also been shown to produce such effects.

Psychiatric disorders, such as depression, anxiety, and withdrawal from substances that depress or alter cerebral functioning, have all been found to affect sleep-wake regulation and functioning. In addition, there is now evidence that links depression, bipolar disorder, and schizophrenia with disordered circadian rhythms, and many of these patients show delayed sleep-wake phase cycle.[5]

OVERVIEW OF DEMENTIA

According to the DSM-5, dementia is a progressive condition or syndrome characterized by memory loss and deficits in other cognitive functions, such as language, problem-solving, and other thinking abilities, that are severe enough to interfere with daily life.[4] The DSM-5 refers to the term dementia as major neurocognitive disorder; the word major in major neurocognitive disorder reveals that the cognitive deficits result in functional impairment, and distinguishes it from mild neurocognitive disorder, which consists of cognitive decline but not significant functional decline.[4]

Cognition is described in the *Oxford Dictionary* as the mental actions or processes involved in acquiring, maintaining, and understanding knowledge through thought, experience, and the senses.[6]

The following are the domains or functions associated with cognition:

- Memory: the encoding (storing) and retrieving (recalling) of memories. Memories can be verbal, visual, or procedural (eg, riding a bike).
- Attention: the ability to focus on a task and shifting to a more relevant stimulus when warranted. Attention is an important component to memory.
- Language: the ability to comprehend and express spoken and written language.
- Visuospatial function: the processing of visual information in space, including identifying objects and where they are.
- Praxis: the ability to perform complex motor tasks (eg, buttoning and unbuttoning clothing).
- Executive function: the ability to process and respond appropriately to incoming information or stimuli.
- Social cognition: the ability to interact with and understand other people, interpreting social cues and appropriately responding to them.

CAUSES OF DEMENTIA

The word dementia is a general term for loss of memory, language, problem-solving, and other cognitive abilities that are severe enough to interfere with daily life. Note that such significant decline in cognition and function is not caused by the normal aging process. Persons living with dementia generally have abnormal brain changes or a neurodegenerative brain disorder, such as Alzheimer's disease (AD), Lewy body dementia (LBD), cerebrovascular disease, frontotemporal dementia (FTD), dementia of Parkinson's disease (PDD), and Huntington disease. Mixed dementia refers to the condition in which brain changes of more than 1 cause of dementia occur simultaneously. **Fig. 2** represents the commonly used umbrella term of dementia and its multiple possible causes.

AD is the most common cause of dementia in older adults, the sixth-leading cause of death in the United States and is the fifth-leading cause of death among those aged 65 years and older. AD, presented in the DSM-5 as Major or Mild Neurocognitive Disorder due to AD, affects memory, language, visuospatial, and executive function, ultimately resulting in a progressive decline in the ability to conduct daily tasks, often referred to as activities of daily living (ADLs).[4]

AD is not a normal part of aging. The greatest known risk factor is increasing age, and most persons living with AD are aged 65 years and older. Note that AD is not just a disease of older adults. Approximately 200,000 Americans less than 65 years of age have younger-onset AD, also known as early-onset AD.[7]

The pathologic hallmarks of AD are amyloid plaques and fibrillary tangles in addition to inflammation.[8] These pathologic changes may begin 20 years or more before symptoms appear, raising the possibility of early identification of persons at risk who may benefit from risk-reduction strategies.

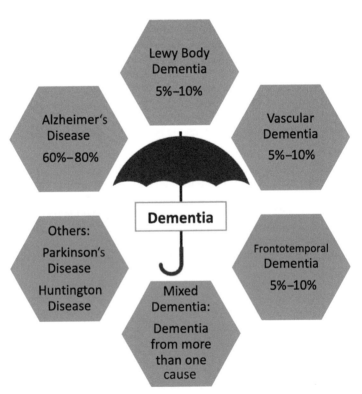

Fig. 2. Types and causes of dementia.

The term Alzheimer's disease and related dementias (ADRD) is used to describe related dementias that are mixtures of different brain disorders that may lead to vascular dementia, LBD, and frontotemporal disorders, to name a few as described earlier, and can be difficult to distinguish clinically from AD.

CARE POINTS

- Dementia is a progressive condition characterized by memory loss and deficits in other cognitive functions, such as language, problem-solving, and other thinking abilities, that are severe enough to interfere with daily life.
- Dementia is an umbrella term covering the types of specific dementias.
- AD is considered 1 type, as well as the most common cause of, dementia and is not a normal part of the aging process.
- ADRD encompasses the types of dementia, including but not limited to AD, LBD, vascular dementia, frontotemporal dementia, and PDD.

PERSON-CENTERED AND FAMILY-CENTERED CARE

Neurocognitive disorders such as ADRD continue to challenge the nation. ADRD cannot be cured, and the ability of medication to delay disease progression is limited. At the same time, the psychosocial burden of ADRD is enormous, affecting patients, their families, and society as a whole. These needs are inadequately addressed by the nation's traditional model of standard health care, the focus of which is primarily biomedical. Person-centered and family-centered care are the foundation for identifying and meeting the needs of individuals through interpersonal relationships that maintain the selfhood of persons living with ADRD (PLWD) and their caregivers.

The Dance of Caring Persons (**Fig. 3**) symbolizes valuing each person while engaging in a rhythm that connects all as guided by the theory of nursing as caring.[9] Each person is in the circle because of their unique contribution to the person and family being cared for.[9]

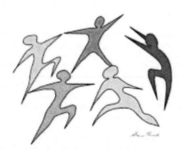

The Dance of Caring Persons

Fig. 3. The dance of caring persons.[10] (Reprinted with permission from A. Boykin & S. O. Schoenhofer (2001, p. 37). Nursing as caring: A model for transforming practice. (1993). New York, NY: National League for Nursing Press.)[10]

SLEEP AND OLDER ADULTS

Older adults are defined as adults aged 65 years or older. In the United States, there is a projected growth of 78 million people between 2017 and 2060. By 2035, it is projected that older adults will outnumber children for the first time in US history.[10] Approximately 50% of older adults complain about difficulty initiating or maintaining sleep. Based on what is known about the limits of self-reported complaints in older adults with ADRD, it can be assumed that this approximation is an underestimation, leaving out the number of older adults who experience the aforementioned sleep disorder symptoms but have not reported them or are unable to do so. "Although sleep disturbance is a common complaint among patients of all ages, research suggests that older adults are particularly vulnerable."[11] As adults age into older adults, marked changes in sleep start to occur. These changes include "an advanced sleep phase and decreased slow-wave sleep, which result in fragmented sleep and early awakening."[11]

Aging is associated with several well-documented changes in sleep-wake patterns, including a tendency to go to sleep earlier in the evenings and wake up earlier in the mornings. Higher instances of waking more frequently during the night and experiencing fragmented sleep have also been reported. "The prevalence of many sleep disorders increases with age."[12]

The circadian process follows the naturally occurring light-dark cycle in the environment. In someone with typical, or normal, functioning, "discrete brain regions promote wakefulness [and] sleep-promoting brain regions, including the anterior hypothalamus and the ventrolateral preoptic nucleus, regulate sleep onset."[13] Because of neurodegeneration that occurs with the aging process, these mechanisms in older adults become less functional and, thus, the circadian rhythm is less able to regulate the sleep-wake cycle.

Epidemiologically, the development of age-related neurodegenerative diseases such as AD and Parkinson's disease is associated with pronounced sleep disruption, whereas emerging mechanistic studies suggest that sleep disruption may be causally linked to neurodegenerative disorder, proposing that sleep may represent a key therapeutic target in the prevention of these conditions.[13]

CARE POINTS

- Aging is associated with several well-documented changes in sleep and in the sleep-wake cycle.
- Because of neurodegeneration during the aging process, these mechanisms in older adults become less functional and, thus, the circadian rhythm is less able to regulate the sleep-wake cycle.

SLEEP AND DEMENTIA

Historically, it has been speculated that memories are processed during sleep. In adults, the evidence shows that good sleep is positively correlated with improved memory recall and a more effective ability of the body to regulate metabolism, reducing mental fatigue.[14] Within the brain, the mechanisms responsible for regulating sleep are also responsible for regulating memory processes. Thus, within an aging brain that develops dementia, these regulatory processes are less functional, leading to adverse effects on memory recall.

There is a known bidirectional relationship between dementia and sleep disturbances; "the bi-directional link of sleep and neurodegenerative disease may influence each other in many ways that have important implications for the diagnosis and treatment of AD"[15] and dementia.[16,17]

Studies have found that sleep disruption and deprivation, resulting in poor sleep quality, are linked to an accumulation of amyloid plaque and tau proteins in the neocortex of the brain, which contribute to the disorder of AD.

As presented by Roth and Brunton,[18] while a person is awake, there is an increase in extracellular levels of metabolites produced by neuronal activity, such as amyloid-β and tau proteins, in the brain. During restorative sleep, these metabolites are cleared from the brain through the glymphatic system.[18] When the sleep-wake cycle is disrupted, clearance of these metabolites is diminished; thus, the accumulation of amyloid-β and tau proteins has been observed to contribute to the forming of amyloid plaques and neurofibrillary tangles characteristically seen in people living with AD.[18]

SLEEP DISORDERS AND FAMILY CAREGIVERS

In 2019, more than 16 million family members and other unpaid caregivers provided an estimated 18.6 billion hours of care to people with ADRD.[19] Nationally, this care is valued at nearly $244 billion, but its costs expand to family caregivers' increased risk for emotional distress and negative mental and physical health outcomes.[19] Of the estimated 10 million adult caregivers of PLWD globally and 4.4 million caregivers nationally, an approximate two-thirds experience sleep disturbance at some point related to their role as caregivers.[20,21]

Accounting for these sleep disturbances and disruptions among caregivers are nighttime behavioral disturbances often seen in PLWD, especially as dementia progresses. Note that research supports the notion that increased difficulty with sleep for both the PLWD and the caregiver is most often linked to a change in living arrangements (eg, the PLWD being placed in a residential facility).

It has been found that caregivers who endure sleep disturbances chronically are consequently more tired during the day; as a result, they can be "more irritable with their care recipient, prone toward household or motor vehicle accidents, and more likely to have difficulty with rapid or complex problem-solving in the face of dementia-related behavioral disturbances."[20,21]

Because quality of life is so affected by quality of sleep for both the PLWD and the family caregiver, both persons' needs should be considered in this regard. Further, because of the link between poor sleep and worsening medical and mental health in all persons, it is critical to ensure that both the PLWD and family caregiver practice good sleep hygiene, maintain an adequate sleep schedule, and get adequate good sleep.

The chronic nature of ADRD contributes significantly to the public health impact related to the illness because much of the time diagnosed is spent in a state of disability, where patients depend on others for their care and support in completing ADLs.[18] In many cases, the brunt of this burden falls on families and caregivers who, as a result, experience emotional stress; depression; new or exacerbated health problems of their own, including physical difficulties and financial challenges; and an overall impact, typically adverse, to their quality of life. Insomnia often emerges or increases among caregivers when the need to provide nighttime care becomes frequent. It has been reported that approximately one-third of family caregivers report that their own health deteriorated after they stepped into the role of being a caregiver.[18]

CARE POINTS

- Sleep disturbances have adverse effects on both the patient and the patient's primary caregiver.
- Because of the bidirectional relationship between sleep patterns and medical and mental health management, sleep should be addressed and managed for both the patient and the patient's caregiver, in order to obtain the best outcomes for both, especially when it comes to the caregiver's ability to care adequately for the patient.

TREATMENT AND MANAGEMENT OF SLEEP DISORDERS

Appropriate treatment should be determined after a comprehensive assessment of symptom severity, comorbidities, and medications already being taken by the patient. Efficacious pharmacologic interventions for sleep disorders in the general population are nonbenzodiazepine hypnotics such as zolpidem, zaleplon, and eszopiclone; ramelteon and immediate-release and modified-release indiplon have also been clinically proved to be effective.[22] Cognitive behavior therapy alone and implemented in conjunction with pharmacologic interventions has been effective in improving sleep in older adults.[22]

The population of older adults is more vulnerable than the general population to adverse side effects and drug interactions that may occur with any pharmacologic agent; therefore, a structured approach should be taken and pharmacologic agents should be introduced after first implementing a nonpharmacologic intervention and with caution.[23] Nonpharmacologic interventions, such as maintaining good sleep hygiene and adequate social and physical activity during the day, may also help to negate instances of sleep-wake disorders.

It has been recommended that, by way of a structured approach, primary sleep disorders such as obstructive sleep apnea be treated first.[23] Subsequently, medications and coexisting conditions that may be affecting a person's sleep or sleep-wake cycle should be assessed and managed.

When assessing risk factors for ADRD, clinicians do not typically focus on sleep as a primary predictor and worsening factor.

TREATMENT AND MANAGEMENT OF SLEEP DISORDERS IN OLDER ADULTS WITH DEMENTIA

Ooms and Ju[24] present a summary of the current recommended clinical approach to sleep disorders in patients living with ADRD. It has been recommended that treatments such as bright light therapy and melatonin supplementation be tried first, before pharmacologic agents, because of the risk of cognitive side effects that are especially plausible among patients living with ADRD. Notable risks have been identified as cognitive side effects, sedation, and falls among the population of older adults and those living with ADRD.[24]

It is emphasized throughout the literature that obtaining an accurate history is crucial, and obtaining collateral information from those close to the patient and involved in the patient's care is critical to that accuracy. Information about sleep patterns, behaviors, and habits should be collected and reported for accurate assessment of the patient's sleep. It is further stressed that any dementia-specific symptoms should be communicated, especially as they relate to the patient's sleeping schedule, patterns, and any sleep-related symptoms.[24]

Mood and anxiety disorder–related symptoms should also be assessed as part of a clinical approach to sleep disorders in dementia because of the overlap of symptoms that can occur and the nature of psychological symptoms that commonly affect sleep; antidepressants, antipsychotics, and other psychiatric drugs should be assessed if being taken by the patient presenting with dementia and sleep disorder–related symptoms in order to rule out contraindications with sleep.[24]

DIAGNOSIS OF SLEEP DISORDERS

Clinical diagnoses of sleep disorders must include obtaining the patient's medical and social history (an important aspect of which is collateral information obtained from the family caregiver, significant other, professional caregiver, and so forth, in PLWD), the patient's self-reports of sleep quality, and the patient's self-reported perception of sleep quality. The clinical diagnosis of insomnia is reached based on a self-reported complaint of trouble falling asleep and/or staying asleep, or early morning awakening, leading to daytime dysfunction. "This daytime dysfunction can manifest in a wide range of ways, including fatigue, malaise; impairment in attention, concentration or memory; impaired social, family, occupational or academic performance; mood disturbance, irritability, sleepiness, hyperactivity, impulsivity, aggression, reduced motivation, proneness for errors, and concerns about or dissatisfaction with sleep."[23] Required for diagnosis, the sleep disturbance must occur within a safe, dark environment, conducive to adequate sleep. Duration and persistence of symptoms are also key to the diagnosis.[24]

Sleep studies are often ordered and implemented in an effort to assess the patient's sleep, during which the patient's total sleep time, sleep latency, slow wave sleep, wake after sleep onset, REM, and NREM sleep are observed and monitored in a controlled setting in order to assess the sleep-wake cycle and patterns that manifest during a night's sleep.[25] "Screening for primary sleep disorders, such as sleep apnea syndrome, restless legs syndrome and rapid eye movement sleep behavior disorder, is essential."[25]

Sleep studies have their limitations, such as testing effects, where the test setting does not capture wholly the naturalistic setting at home, as do self-reported data collected through clinical intake interviewing, so clinicians must do the most comprehensive assessment possible, combining all objective and subjective data to rule out differential diagnoses, such as insomnia, in favor of a sleep-wake disorder diagnosis. During sleep studies, the examinee is connected via wires to the testing equipment; this alone may cause anxiety or worry, especially in PLWD, but it may also impede physical comfort, necessary to fall asleep or stay asleep. Further, research has strongly supported the idea that PLWD can become agitated and/or confused in any setting or environment that is unfamiliar to them, which could also affect the execution and results of a sleep study.[26] "Individuals with ADRD are at risk of developing delirium and experiencing stress related to an unfamiliar environment."[26]

It is worth mentioning again that it is critical to obtain reports from the caregiver caring for the PLWD with regard to the patient's sleep, to provide details, and to corroborate details provided by the patient, if applicable, in order to fully capture the picture of how sleep is being managed, or not, at home.

SLEEP DISORDER DIAGNOSIS AND COMORBIDITIES

Note the overlap that often exists between sleep disorder symptoms and the presence of another disorder, especially depression, anxiety, or another psychological disorder that may better explain the sleep disturbance; clinicians may offer a dual diagnosis or may favor 1 more than the other, based on the disorder or illness the symptoms best describe. In 1 review, a staggering number of individuals who present with depressive symptoms had sought independent specialized medical treatment of sleep disturbances or issues, "which raises the unsettling possibility that many cases of depression go undetected."[27]

If older adults present with appetite loss, fatigue, lethargy, and loss of appetite, they may meet the clinical diagnostic criteria for depression; if this is the case, when treated, a lessening the severity of sleep-related symptoms may occur.

SLEEP DISORDER DIAGNOSIS IN PERSONS LIVING WITH DEMENTIA

The biological mechanisms responsible for the biological processes related to maintaining adequate sleep become less effective with age. Especially for older adults with ADRD, the sleep-wake pattern is often a prerequisite for the best possible quality of life and the best health outcomes. In older adults, a lower homeostatic sleep pressure decreases the amount of slow-wave sleep.[28]

More than 60% of persons had 1 or more sleep disturbances, almost invariably associated one to another without any evident and specific pattern of co-occurrence. Persons with AD and those with mild cognitive impairment (MCI) had the same frequency of any sleep disorder. Sleep-disordered breathing was more frequent in vascular dementia. REM behavior disorder was more represented in LBD or PDD.[28]

The prevalence of sleep disturbances increasing with age suggests that sleep is affected by aging itself and/or by aging-related conditions. Sleep disturbances are particularly frequent in persons with dementia or cognitive impairment. The high prevalence of sleep disorders reported in neurodegenerative diseases could be explained by intrinsic changes specific to each form of dementia but also by the high prevalence of other generalized conditions potentially affecting sleep and the sleep-wake cycle in these persons. Such conditions include depression, chronic pain, use of medications causing side effects, and low levels of cognitive and physical activity or stimulation. Further, sleep can be affected by neurologic changes that affect a person's circadian rhythm: it is highly plausible that the diffuse brain damage that characterizes dementias might extend over the cognitive brain areas to involve the neural networks that control sleep function (anterior hypothalamus, reticular activating system, suprachiasmatic nucleus, and pineal gland). Sleep disorders seem to be different in each form of dementia, and this might be the consequence of the different brain pathologic involvement that characterizes each dementia type.[28]

In terms of the coexistence and comorbidity of sleep disorders with other dementias, OSA is seen at high rates among patients with vascular dementia or vascular cognitive impairment, and it has been postulated that the presence of sleep disturbances in a person presenting with MCI increases the risk of MCI developing or evolving into ADRD.[28]

Assessment of sleep and circadian disturbances in dementia begins with a complete history. Because persons living with ADRD may not recall symptoms accurately, collateral history from caregivers is essential. The clinical history should assess for symptoms of primary sleep disorders, such as snoring, hypersomnia, witnessed apneas, parasomnias, restless legs, and leg movements during sleep. The timing and regularity of nighttime sleep and daytime naps (intentional and inadvertent) are important to ascertain. In addition to these clinical features typically queried during a sleep evaluation, individuals with dementia should be specifically asked about sundowning, hallucinations, sleep attacks, injurious parasomnias, and nighttime wandering. If the cause of dementia is known, the history should query for sleep-wake problems characteristic of the underlying disease. For example, in someone with Parkinson's disease, a detailed temporal relationship between dopaminergic medication dosing and restless legs syndrome symptoms should be obtained. In all cases, the overall burden of sleep disturbances on both patient and caregiver should be considered. Sleep and circadian rhythm disturbances that negatively affect sleep quality can negatively affect the quality of life of both the patient and the caregiver, worsening health outcomes for each.[24]

Contributory factors should be assessed, including but not limited to depression, anxiety, and mood disorder symptoms or diagnoses; comorbidities relating to physical pain and discomfort; other comorbidities; medications, including supplements and over-the-counter medications; alcohol and caffeine consumption; drug and tobacco use; environmental factors; sleep patterns and environment; living arrangements; social engagement and interaction; physical activity; and nutrition. Scales such as the Epworth Sleepiness Scale or Pittsburgh Sleep Quality Index, although they have not been validated specifically for use in patients with dementia, have been found to be useful in identifying trends over time and, in conjunction with self-reported data and collateral information by a caregiver, may aid clinicians in assessing and managing the sleep disorder symptoms.[24]

CARE POINTS

- Sleep-wake cycle disturbances are common in AD and LBD.
- Sleep disturbances in persons living with ADRD (PLWD) can negatively affect the health of the caregiver.
- Nighttime awakenings by PLWD are a common precipitating factor of sleep-wake disturbances in caregivers.
- The high prevalence and consequences of insomnia in PLWD necessitate a comprehensive medical and psychosocial evaluation, including sleep history.
- The caregivers or family members should be included in the evaluation of PLWD in order to obtain an accurate history and to identify and address the unique needs of the caregivers.

SLEEP DISTURBANCE AND BEHAVIORAL AND PSYCHOLOGICAL SYMPTOMS OF DEMENTIA

A disordered sleep-wake cycle has many implications for older adults living with ADRD. For example, vascular events such as a chronic obstruction of oxygen flow to the brain can lead to and exacerbate neurocognitive decline related to the neurocognitive disorders. Further, even if unrelated directly to poor sleep quality, older adults with ADRD who do not have a well-reinforced sleep-wake cycle often present with sundowning, a condition named for and marked by a characteristic exacerbation of behavioral and psychological symptoms of dementia (BPSD) as the sun goes down and the day comes to an end. Although the cause of sundowning is not exactly understood, it is thought to be related to an adversely affected circadian rhythm (ie, the brain's inability to process time, which worsens over time across the course of the ADRD progression); "reduced circadian signals in the elderly result in reduced core body temperature and a phase advance of wake and sleep times."[25] The research supports that some effective strategies to manage sundowning include adherence to a healthy sleep-wake cycle, exposing the patient to sunlight or artificial lighting during the day, and maintaining a well-lit environment for the patient until it is time to go to bed.[24,25] These strategies support the importance of PLWD obtaining adequate sleep of good quality, as a maintenance strategy for overall quality of life, for both the patients and the caregivers.

Studies have found that approximately 90% of persons living with ADRD experience behavioral and psychological symptoms, referred to as BPSD.[29] BPSD are prevalent and can considerably affect the prognosis and management of dementia. For this reason, the DSM-5 requires clinicians to specify whether BPSD are present and to indicate the degree of severity; for example, a diagnosis of dementia caused by AD might be coded as a major neurocognitive disorder caused by AD, with behavioral disturbances, severe.

Sleep disorders caused by REM sleep behavior is one of the most common BPSD. Others include depression, delusions, hallucinations, agitation, verbal and physical aggression, anxiety, irritability, disinhibition, restlessness, wondering, changes in eating, and refusal of care and taking medications. Sleep disturbances are common in ADRD, especially AD and LBD.

Sleep disorders in persons living with ADRD not only affect the person with the disease but they significantly contribute to the physical and psychological burden family caregivers experience. This issue was discussed earlier in relation to sleep disorders and family caregivers.

CARE POINTS

- Evidence-based strategies found to be effective in managing sundowning include adherence to a healthy sleep-wake cycle, exposing the patient to sunlight or artificial lighting during the day, and maintaining a well-lit environment for the patient until it is time to go to bed.
- It is important that people living with ADRD obtain adequate sleep of good quality.
- Maintaining healthy sleep hygiene for people living with ADRD has mutual benefits for their quality of life and the quality of life of the caregivers.

INSOMNIA IN OLDER ADULTS AND OLDER ADULTS WITH ALZHEIMER'S DISEASE AND RELATED DEMENTIAS

One of the most commonly occurring sleep disturbances in the population of older adults is insomnia. It is estimated that more than 50% of older adults complain about difficulty initiating or maintaining sleep.[30] Note that this approximation cannot include older adults who have difficulty self-reporting their symptoms, namely those experiencing declining cognitive functioning and trouble with self-expression. Because the aforementioned obstacles are often present for PLWD, the authors emphasize the need of an advocate, usually the primary caregiver, to recognize and report symptoms of sleep disturbance in PLWD who may otherwise not be able to report them themselves.

PLWD often undergo a shift in their sleep-wake cycles, experiencing insomnia during the night, waking up often, and having difficulty staying asleep, and also napping during the daytime, which exacerbates the sleep disturbance cycle. In the late stages of AD, people may have a complete reversal of the usual daytime wakefulness and nighttime sleep pattern.

REFLECTIONS AND FUTURE DIRECTIONS
Optimizing Care

The importance of accurate and timely diagnosis to identify sleep-wake disturbances in persons living with ADRD must be emphasized through a comprehensive clinical evaluation in order to optimize care and improve health outcomes. Clinicians should focus on identifying sleep-wake disturbances in PLWD, diagnose the probable cause of the dementia, as well as addressing and managing sleep disturbances detected in the caregiver. A person-centered and family-centered approach ought to be integrated as a guiding principle while evaluating and providing care for PLWD and their caregivers if improved patient outcomes are desired. Older adults of ethnic and other diverse populations, such as those from the Lesbian, Gay, Bisexual, Transgender, Queer and/or Questioning (LGBTQ) community, face barriers to dementia-specific care and supportive services, resulting in cognitive and overall decline. Culturally and linguistically appropriate care is part of person-centered care and best practice.

Challenges

Considering the weak contemporary evidence regarding the efficacy of pharmacologic interventions for sleep disturbances in PLWD, nonpharmacologic approaches, including psychological, behavioral, and environmental interventions, should be considered as the first line of treatment. This recommendation, even though safest to adopt, poses challenges because of the lack of standardization as a result of the many variables each person presents in terms of overall health and response to treatment, in addition to the changing trajectory of the disease.

RESEARCH: DIVERSITY AND INCLUSIVITY

Walasezek (2020)[31] explains that the effects of nonpharmacologic approaches in PLWD have been studied mostly in long-term care settings, thus results cannot appropriately be applied to community-dwelling older adults living with ADRD. Research in this area is needed to be conducted in the patients' own homes. Furthermore, recruitment into clinical trials should include the older and frailer segments of the elderly population, such as those living with ADRD. Recruitment of elderly ethnic and other diverse populations into clinical trials should also be expanded. Persons who identify themselves as being LGBTQ, and their caregivers, should be cared for within an inclusive environment. Research is needed on multiple levels (molecular, cellular, system, population) to clarify the effect of race and ethnicity on disease prevalence and on variations in the effectiveness of pharmacologic and nonpharmacologic interventions for sleep disorders in PLWD.

DISCLOSURE STATEMENT

Dr. María de los Ángeles Ordóñez: served as consultant for Eisai Inc. Advisory Board, with a focus on APRN's role in diagnosing patients with AD; she recently became aware that this company manufactures medications for the treatment of insomnia. Medications mentioned in the article were chosen without knowledge of any association with this company.

Patricia de los Ángeles Ordóñez: nothing to disclose.

REFERENCES

1. Insufficient sleep is a public health problem. Cdc.gov; 2017. Available at: https://www.cdc.gov/sleep/data_statistics.html. Accessed March 23, 2021.

2. Roth T. Insomnia: definition, prevalence, etiology, and consequences. J Clin Sleep Med 2007;3(5 Suppl):S7–10.
3. Statista Research Department. Common sleep problems among adults U.S. by age 2017. 2019. Available at: https://www.statista.com/statistics/668080/common-sleep-issues-among-us-adults-age/. Accessed November 9, 2020.
4. American Psychiatric Association. Diagnostic and statistical manual of mental disorders. 5th edition. American Psychiatric Publishing; 2013.
5. Ohayon MM. Prevalence and comorbidity of sleep disorders in general population. Rev Prat 2007;57(14):1521–8.
6. Cognition. Available at: Oxfordreference.com. Accessed November 9, 2020.
7. Alzheimer's Association. 2018 Alzheimer's disease facts and figures. Alz.org; 2018. Available at: https://www.alz.org/media/documents/facts-and-figures-2018-r.pdf. Accessed November 10, 2020.
8. Sperling RA, Aisen PS, Beckett LA, et al. Toward defining the preclinical stages of Alzheimer's disease: recommendations from the National Institute on Aging-Alzheimer's Association workgroups on diagnostic guidelines for Alzheimer's disease. Alzheimers Dement 2011;7(3):280–92.
9. Boykin A, Schoenhofer S. The role of nursing leadership in creating caring environments in health care delivery systems. Nurs Adm Q 2001;25(3):1–7.
10. Population Estimates and Projections. Demographic turning points for the united States: Population projections for 2020 to 2060. Census.gov. Available at: https://www.census.gov/content/dam/Census/library/publications/2020/demo/p25-1144.pdf. Accessed November 10, 2020.
11. Roepke SK, Ancoli-Israel S. Sleep disorders in the elderly. Indian J Med Res 2010;131:302–10.
12. Suzuki K, Miyamoto M, Hirata K. Sleep disorders in the elderly: diagnosis and management 2017. Available at: https://www.ncbi.nlm.nih.gov/pmc/articles/PMC5689397/. Accessed August 24, 2020.
13. Wolkove N, Elkholy O, Baltzan M, et al. Sleep and aging: 1. Sleep disorders commonly found in older people. CMAJ 2007;176(9):1299e304.
14. Bah T, Goodman J, Iliff J. Sleep as a therapeutic target in the aging brain. Neurotherapeutics 2019;16(3):554–68.
15. Eugene AR, Masiak J. The neuroprotective aspects of sleep 2015. Available at: https://www.ncbi.nlm.nih.gov/pmc/articles/PMC4651462/. Accessed November 14, 2020.
16. Vaou OE, Lin SH, Branson C, et al. Sleep and dementia. Curr Sleep Med Rep 2018;4(2):134–42.
17. Wu M, Rosenberg P, Spira A, et al. Sleep disturbance, cognitive decline, and dementia: a review. Semin Neurol 2017;37(04):395–406.
18. Roth T, Brunton S. Identification and management of insomnia in Alzheimer's disease. J Fam Pract 2019;68(8):S32–8.
19. 2020 Alzheimer's disease facts and figures. Alzheimers Dement 2020;16(3):391–460.
20. McCurry SM, Logsdon RG, Teri L, et al. Sleep disturbances in caregivers of persons with dementia: contributing factors and treatment implications. Sleep Med Rev 2007;11(2):143–53.
21. Ancoli-Israel S. Sleep and aging: prevalence of disturbed sleep and treatment considerations in older adults. J Clin Psychiatry 2005;66(Suppl 9):24–30 [quiz 42-3].

22. Ancoli-Israel S, Kripke DF, Mason W, et al. Comparisons of home sleep recordings and polysomnograms in older adults with sleep disorders. Sleep 1981; 4(3):283–91.
23. Krystal AD, Prather AA, Ashbrook LH. The assessment and management of insomnia: an update. World Psychiatry 2019;18(3):337–52.
24. Ooms S, Ju Y-E. Treatment of sleep disorders in dementia. Curr Treat Options Neurol 2016;18(9):40.
25. Suzuki K, Miyamoto M, Hirata K. Sleep disorders in the elderly: diagnosis and management. J Gen Fam Med 2017;18(2):61–71.
26. Holden TR, Keller S, Kim A, et al. Procedural framework to facilitate hospital-based informed consent for dementia research. J Am Geriatr Soc 2018;66(12): 2243–8.
27. Ohayon MM, Caulet M, Lemoine P. Comorbidity of mental and insomnia disorders in the general population. Compr Psychiatry 1998;39(4):185–97.
28. Guarnieri B, Adorni F, Musicco M, et al. Prevalence of sleep disturbances in mild cognitive impairment and dementing disorders: a multicenter Italian clinical cross-sectional study on 431 patients. Dement Geriatr Cogn Disord 2012; 33(1):50–8.
29. Müller-Spahn F. Behavioral disturbances in dementia. Dialogues Clin Neurosci 2003;5(1):49–59.
30. Patel D, Steinberg J, Patel P. Insomnia in the elderly: a review. J Clin Sleep Med 2018;14(6):1017–24.
31. Walaszek A, editor. Behavioral and psychological symptoms of dementia. American Psychiatric Association Publishing; 2019.

Clinical Decision-Making

Restless Legs Syndrome and Dementia in Older Adults

Kathy Richards, PhD, RN[a], Katherine Carroll Britt, BSN, RN[b],
Norma Cuellar, PhD, RN[c],*, Yanyan Wang, PhD[b],
Janet Morrison, PhD, RN[b]

KEYWORDS

- Restless legs syndrome • Alzheimer disease • Dementia • Sleep • Agitation

KEY POINTS

- Older adults with dementia are at high risk for having undiagnosed RLS.
- Many commonly prescribed medications exacerbate RLS symptoms; therefore, it is important to consider deprescribing.
- RLS signs in this population may include sleep disturbances, wandering, rubbing the legs, and an inability to sit still during the evening and first half of the night.
- There is a low evidence base for RLS treatment in dementia patients warranting more clinical trials.
- A thorough evaluation is the first step and treatment should focus on relieving discomfort while identifying and treating worrisome sleep symptoms.

INTRODUCTION

In older adults with dementia, sleep disturbances are highly prevalent. Approximately 45% to 55% of older adults with dementia have sleep disturbances that adversely impact their cognitive functioning and quality of life[1,2]; increase caregiver burden; and often result in more restrictive levels of care, such as admission to long-term care facilities.[3,4] Clinical decision-making in older adults with multiple chronic health conditions is challenging, especially in patients with dementing illnesses who are unable cognitively or verbally to describe their symptoms and responses to interventions. In this article, we discuss clinical decision-making in older adults with

[a] The University of Texas at Austin, School of Nursing, 1710 Red River Street, Austin, TX 78712, USA; [b] The University of Texas at Austin, School of Nursing, 1712 Red River Street, Austin, TX 78712, USA; [c] The University of Alabama, University Boulevard, 650 University Boulevard East, Tuscaloosa, AL 35401, USA
* Corresponding author.
E-mail address: ncuellar@ua.edu
Twitter: @kathyrichards2 (K.R.); @KatherineCBritt1 (K.C.B.); @NormaCuellar61 (N.C.); @yanw06689982 (Y.W.); @phdb4ss (J.M.)

Nurs Clin N Am 56 (2021) 265–274
https://doi.org/10.1016/j.cnur.2021.02.005
0029-6465/21/© 2021 Elsevier Inc. All rights reserved.

nursing.theclinics.com

dementia and restless legs syndrome (RLS), one of the more prevalent sleep disturbances.

RLS occurs in approximately 1 in 10 Americans, with a higher prevalence in older adults.[5] Also called Willis-Ekbom disease, RLS is best known for irresistible and unpleasant urges to move the legs during the early part of the night while at rest, interfering with sleep onset and maintenance. It is often underdiagnosed or misdiagnosed in older adults with dementing illnesses, who frequently cannot reliably self-report RLS sleep-related symptoms.[6,7] Once RLS is diagnosed, however, implementation of treatment effectively relieves discomfort and improves sleep quality, both of which are health priorities for older adults regardless of their health trajectories. The article provides an overview of RLS, describes sleep disturbances in older adults with RLS and dementia, discusses assessment of RLS in this population, identifies non-pharmacologic and pharmacologic interventions, and communicates key clinical decision-making recommendations.

OVERVIEW OF RESTLESS LEGS SYNDROME

RLS is a complex neurologic disorder that affects movement and sleep, consisting of uncomfortable neurosensory sensations that prompt limb movements and thus disrupt patients' sleep and their ability to function in daily life.[8–14] Walking typically relieves RLS symptoms, such that RLS sufferers are often referred to as "night walkers." An RLS diagnosis arises from patients' self-reports of the following clinical features: (1) a forceful urge to move the legs,[15–17] often accompanied by sensations that patients describe as painful, electrical, prickling, burning, tingling, and/or itching[18,19]; (2) improvement of symptoms following voluntary movement or involuntary periodic limb movements; (3) a worsening of symptoms during periods of inactivity; and (4) a peak in symptoms at night.[20–22] In addition, these features are not caused by any other medical or behavioral condition.[23] This subjective urge to move with relief of symptoms through movement is especially characteristic of RLS. Patients also seek treatment of associated sleep disruptions. Clinical severity is judged by the number of days per week with symptoms, the time of onset during the day, and the number of leg movements that occur during sleep.

Sleep-onset latency (difficulty falling asleep) and sleep fragmentation are commonly reported in RLS and can lead to serious, sometimes disabling, disturbance of daytime functioning.[20–22,24] The exact pathophysiology of RLS is unclear, but dopamine and iron metabolism dysfunction are strongly implicated.[25,26] The clinical course of RLS suggests that two forms exist: primary and secondary, yet symptoms of both do not differ in presentation or treatment. Primary or idiopathic RLS tends to first occur early in life and is largely genetic, whereas secondary RLS arises later in life alongside chronic health conditions (eg, renal disease, pregnancy, heart disease, and diabetes).[9,23,27,28] Secondary RLS has a steeper progression, with more severe symptoms, more patient distress, and worse life disruption.[11,28,29] RLS is a progressive disorder that worsens with age, and it is more prevalent in Europeans and North Americans. It is more common in females, with a prevalence of 5.0% in men (range, 2%–9.4%) and 8.8% in women (range, 2.3%–15.4%).[30] A systematic review[5] found a prevalence of about 12% in European and North American women age 70 to 90 years, a group often affected by comorbid dementia.

RESTLESS LEGS SYNDROME IN OLDER ADULTS WITH DEMENTIA

Characteristics common in persons with dementia are implicated in the metabolic and functional pathways that contribute to RLS, lending support to an increased expression of RLS in this population: older age[31]; female gender[5]; iron deficiency and anemia[32]; vascular causes for dementia, such as stroke[33]; and the frequent use of medications that may aggravate RLS symptoms, such as antinausea drugs (eg, prochlorperazine), serotonin-elevating antidepressants (eg, fluoxetine), antipsychotic drugs (eg, haloperidol), and allergy and cold medications containing older antihistamines (eg, diphenhydramine).[34] A Department of Veterans Affairs–funded study[7] combined several sources of data to diagnose RLS, including caregiver interviews, medical history, iron status, polysomnography with periodic leg movements, direct observation for RLS-associated behaviors, and consensus of expert diagnosticians. These diagnostic methods were applied to 59 older adults with nighttime agitation and dementia living at home; 25% had RLS, which was associated with frequency of nighttime agitation behaviors ($r = 0.31$; $P < .01$). Yet Talarico and colleagues[35] reported a much lower 4.1% prevalence of RLS among 393 patients with mild Alzheimer disease, which they attributed to missing data and the requirement that the patient with dementia complete an RLS survey.

Untreated RLS has serious ramifications for older adults with dementia, including discomfort or pain, nighttime agitation, disturbed sleep, falls, reduced quality of life, and burdened caregivers. Unidentified RLS may be the cause of nighttime agitation in some patients. Commonly known as "sundowning," nighttime agitation is a behavioral state exhibited in the evening and nighttime characterized by wandering and aggression. More than half of persons with dementia experience nighttime agitation, which results in patient suffering, burdened caregivers, and costly management. The circadian patterns of RLS symptoms and nighttime agitation behaviors are nearly indistinguishable.[36]

Although the urge to move in RLS may manifest as wandering or pacing, physical limitations in frail older adults often preclude independent physical mobility. RLS may be exhibited as other behaviors aimed at relieving discomfort, such as general restlessness or cries for help in patients who lack mobility. Multiple awakenings and nighttime wanderings related to RLS can lead to falls, and various medications to treat sleep disturbances and other chronic age-related health conditions can increase falls still more.[6] Furthermore, the extended bedrest during hospitalization and the immobility caused by other chronic health conditions, such as arthritis or heart failure, may exacerbate RLS symptoms.

CLINICAL ASSESSMENT

Clinical assessment of any suspected sleep problem in older adults with dementia should include a global geriatric approach and a tailored clinical decision-making plan based on the patient's health priorities and health trajectory. Features and causes for any sleep problem need to be examined carefully. It is critical to obtain a thorough history from all possible sources, including patients (if able), family members, and formal and informal caregivers. In the nursing home setting, caregivers who consistently care for specific nursing home residents on evening and night shifts can provide information on each resident's usual bedtime, nighttime routines, and quality and quantity of nighttime sleep.[37] For example, a caregiver's report of a patient's early preferred bedtime, immediate falling asleep, few awakenings, and final morning awakening at about 4 AM is not indicative of RLS. However, if a caregiver reports excessive walking during the first half of the night and a delayed bedtime, followed by sleeping soundly during the last half of the night and into the morning, the patient may have RLS. Daytime staff can provide data on the effect of nighttime sleep disturbances on daytime quality-of-life indicators, such as excessive daytime napping, lack of engagement in activities, and sleepiness. In addition to typical inquiries of timing, duration, and regularity of sleep, daytime napping, and specific symptoms, the clinical assessment of sleep in this population should always consider common sleep-disturbing factors in older adults, such as nocturia, respiratory distress, alcohol, pain, depression, light exposure, noise, decreased social and physical activity, and medication use.

Older adults with dementia often cannot recall or describe their specific RLS symptoms.[6] In patients with intact cognition, a verbal report of a circadian variation of urgency to move the legs, with uncomfortable and unpleasant sensations in the legs followed by partial or total relief with movement, is essential for RLS diagnosis.[23] In patients with dementia, however, impaired cognition and communication distort their descriptions of essential diagnostic criteria. The Behavioral Indicators Test–Restless Legs is a validated instrument, consisting of 20-minute structured behavioral observations and clinical indicators for diagnosing RLS in older adults with dementia.[38]

NONPHARMACOLOGIC AND PHARMACOLOGIC INTERVENTIONS

Clinical decision-making regarding treatment of RLS in older adults with dementia should involve collaboration with family members, caregivers, and the older adult (if possible). The overall focus should be on relieving discomfort and identifying and treating troublesome sleep symptoms, such as excessive daytime sleepiness or insufficient nighttime sleep, which negatively affect quality of life for the older adult or increase caregiver burden. As an example, discomfort from RLS may increase nighttime agitation and prompt more restraining care for patient safety.[36] A thorough evaluation is an essential first step if RLS is suspected, followed by treatment of comorbidities or deprescribing medications that may worsen symptoms.

In light of potential adverse side effects of medications, nonpharmacologic interventions are preferred if treatment of comorbidities or deprescribing is not effective. Unfortunately, there is insufficient evidence on the efficacy of nonpharmacologic interventions for RLS, and, to our knowledge, no studies have been conducted in older adults with dementia. One interesting intervention is the Vibratory Counterstimulus Device, which has been approved for RLS treatment by the Food and Drug Administration. In a group receiving treatment with the vibrating pad, in comparison with sham treatment, sleep was found to be significantly improved (N = 158 adults with moderate to severe RLS)[39,40]; however, lack of insurance coverage has been a barrier to uptake. In another randomized pilot controlled trial (N = 28 adults with RLS), a significant decrease in RLS severity ($P = .017$) and a significant improvement in sleep ($P = .005$) were found for participants who received treatment with an MMF07 foot massager (no heat), a device with a motion footplate that moves the feet and legs in a circle, creating a vibrating sensation. In a randomized, double-blinded, sham-controlled trial using a pneumatic compression device in adults with RLS,[41] a decrease in RLS severity ($P = .006$) and an improvement in sleep quality ($P = .05$) were found in those using a pneumatic compression device as opposed to a sham device. In another trial conducted over 12 weeks in adults with RLS (N = 41), lower body resistance and aerobic exercise decreased RLS severity.[42] Other nonpharmacologic interventions for RLS that require further testing include Longden counterstrain manipulation,[43] yoga,[44] and local cryotherapy.[45] Additional high-quality randomized controlled trials are needed to further test the efficacy of nonpharmacologic interventions.

Pharmacologic interventions for RLS in older adults with Alzheimer disease and related dementias should always begin with the deprescribing of medications beginning with gradual tapering and discontinuation if possible. Medications that worsen RLS symptoms or cause adverse events, such as daytime sedation, include: antinausea drugs (eg, prochlorperazine or metoclopramide), antipsychotic drugs (eg, haloperidol or pheno-thiazine derivatives) that cause dopamine antagonism, antidepressants that increase serotonin (eg, fluoxetine or sertraline), and some cold and allergy medications that contain older antihistamines (eg, diphenhydramine).[34] For patients with depression and RLS, substituting bupropion for antidepressants that increase serotonin may improve RLS symptoms.[33]

For patients with sleep disturbances, wandering, other agitation behaviors, and signs of RLS, a trial of pharmacologic treatment of RLS may be indicated. Because of the common co-occurrence of RLS and iron deficiency, an iron panel (ferritin, percent transferrin saturation, total iron binding capacity, and iron) should be checked.[33] For ferritin levels less than 75 ng/mL, clinicians should consider prescribing 325 mg ferrous sulfate by mouth.

Dopamine agonists and alpha-2-delta ligands ($\alpha_2\delta$) are generally considered first-line treatment of RLS.[46] However, dopamine agonists and carbidopa/levodopa are generally not well tolerated in the older adult with dementia. The $\alpha_2\delta$ gabapentin enacarbil is approved by the Food and Drug Administration for treating RLS and has a favorable safety profile and efficacy. The mechanism for the effect of $\alpha_2\delta$ ligands on RLS is thought to be their effect on presynaptic glutamatergic transmission.[47] A growing body of literature links brain iron deficiency, altered glutamatergic transmission, and RLS.

This discussion would be incomplete without mentioning the many medications often prescribed for older adults with multiple chronic health conditions that exacerbate and/or cause sleep disruption. These common medication classes include neuroleptics, antidepressants, antihistamines, proton pump inhibitors, and antiemetics with dopamine blockage.[36] Among residents in nursing homes, older adults with dementing illnesses are exceptionally vulnerable to the pervasiveness of polypharmacy. In a study involving 30,702 residents,[48] the average number of medications was 7%, and 21% of the residents were prescribed 10 or more. Sleep disturbances are often a side effect of medication, and, if unrecognized, they can lead to a surge in prescriptions, further increasing the risk of adverse drug reactions.

EVALUATION

Formal and informal caregivers of older adults with dementia can evaluate treatment response based on their global impressions of change and their observations of improvement in patients' behaviors that may indicate discomfort from RLS, such as rubbing the legs or inability to sit still in the evening and early part of the night, nighttime sleep duration and awakenings, daytime sleepiness, and frequency of nighttime agitation behaviors. They may also consider changes in caregiver burden, caregiver sleep, and patient quality of life. Home caregivers might collect nightly data on RLS signs of discomfort, such as rubbing legs, wandering and pacing behaviors, and sleep

---

Box 1
Clinical care points

- Involve patient, caregivers, and family members in evaluation and treatment
- Consider common sleep-disturbing factors first
- Beware of polypharmacy; deprescribe medications if possible
- Use a sleep diary for compiling observations

Box 2
Case study 1

Alice, a 75-year-old woman with moderate to severe Alzheimer disease, lives at home with her husband of 50 years. James, her husband, reports that her memory is worsening. Lately, she wanders from room to room and repeatedly tries to open the outside doors to get out of the house. A few weeks earlier he forgot to lock one of the doors, and she left their home. Fortunately, the police found her at a nearby shopping center. These wandering and exiting behaviors are more frequent in the evenings, and sometimes continue until 1–2 AM. She has a history of iron deficiency and recently began receiving a selective serotonin reuptake inhibitor for depression. Their 40-year-old daughter has severe RLS. What may be causing these symptoms in Alice?

A. Insomnia

B. Restless legs syndrome

C. Depression

D. Alpha-2-delta ligand medications

Answer: B. RLS is the most likely diagnosis because: movement relieves RLS discomfort, older adults may be phase advanced, including their RLS symptoms. Her behaviors indicate that she may have leg discomfort, family history of RLS, and history of iron deficiency, and selective serotonin reuptake inhibitors may exacerbate RLS symptoms.

Box 3
Case study 2

Peter is an 84-year-old man diagnosed with Lewy body dementia and end-stage renal disease. He lives in an assisted-living facility and is of European descent. He takes sertraline (Zoloft) to manage his depression. In early evening, staff have noted that he is unable to sit still, frequently rubs his legs together in a patterned movement, and displays agitated behavior. His nighttime nurse becomes concerned. What are the next steps the clinical staff should take to evaluate Peter for RLS?

Answer: A thorough evaluation of Peter's behavior is warranted. A sleep diary is a good way to keep track of Peter's sleep patterns and behavior including speaking with nighttime staff about nighttime activity and with family members to learn more about his history. Staff should note any risk factors or contributors to his behavior. Screening for iron deficiency is important, as is considering deprescribing any contributing medications.

Peter's risk factors include European descent, antidepressant medication, older adult, and end-stage renal disease. His iron levels were found to be insufficient and he was started on oral ferrous sulfate. His medication was changed from sertraline to bupropion (Wellbutrin) for his depression.

quality, using a sleep diary. It is highly important to note any side effects of treatments in the diary, such as falls, sedation, or worsening mood, and adherence and tolerance for any nonpharmacologic treatments. **Box 1** provides clinical care points that address evidence-based RLS and dementia recommendations; **Boxes 2** and **3** present Case Studies 1 and 2.

SUMMARY

RLS is a sleep disorder characterized by irresistible and unpleasant urges to move the legs during the early part of the night while at rest, which interferes with sleep. Its prevalence increases with age, with chronic health conditions (eg, diabetes and iron deficiency), and in people of European and Northern American origin; older adults with dementia are at high risk for having the disease but may not be able to report it. Furthermore, medications commonly prescribed for older adults with dementia, such as serotonin reuptake inhibitors for depression, exacerbate RLS symptoms and discomfort. Signs that may indicate RLS in older adults with dementia are sleep disturbances and wandering, rubbing the legs, and inability to sit still during the evening and first half of the night. The Behavioral Indicators Test–Restless Legs is a validated RLS diagnostic tool for older adults with dementia.[38]

Clinical decision-making regarding treatment of RLS in older adults with dementia should involve collaboration among family members, caregivers, and the older adult if possible. The evidence base for treatment in frail older adults is limited. Clinical management decisions should be framed within the context of harms, burdens, benefits, and quality of life. The overall focus of treatment is often on relieving discomfort and identifying and treating troublesome sleep symptoms, such as excessive daytime sleepiness or insufficient nighttime sleep, which negatively affect quality of life for the older adult or increase caregiver burden. As an example, discomfort from RLS may increase nighttime agitation and prompt more restraining care levels for patient safety. A thorough evaluation is an essential first step if RLS is suspected. Treatment of comorbidities that may worsen symptoms, such as iron deficiency, if the risk/benefit ratio is acceptable, and deprescribing of medications that exacerbate RLS symptoms should always be the guiding principles of care. Substitution of medications known to successfully treat RLS but not typically considered in the treatment of dementia-related sleep disturbances (eg, $\alpha_2\delta$ ligands) might be considered when clinical and behavioral indicators of RLS are present.

Additional rigorous clinical trials are needed to identify the most effective nonpharmacologic treatments for RLS. Advocacy for families, regulatory agencies, and professionals is needed to support reimbursement for effective nonpharmacologic interventions. Dedicated rigorous studies of medications in frail older adults are needed to examine their effectiveness and side effects.

DISCLOSURE

Dr K. Richard's research is supported by the National Institutes of Health and Arbor Pharmaceuticals for gabapentin enacarbil and placebo. Additional authors have nothing to disclose.

REFERENCES

1. Zhou G, Liu S, Yu X, et al. High prevalence of sleep disorders and behavioral and psychological symptoms of dementia in late-onset Alzheimer disease: a study in Eastern China. Medicine 2019;98(50):e18405.

2. Moran M, Lynch CA, Walsh C, et al. Sleep disturbance in mild to moderate Alzheimer's disease. Sleep Med 2005;6(4):347–52.
3. Kim SS, Oh KM, Richards K. Sleep disturbance, nocturnal agitation behaviors, and medical comorbidity in older adults with dementia: relationship to reported caregiver burden. Res Gerontol Nurs 2014;7(6):206–14.
4. Gehrman P, Gooneratne NS, Brewster GS, et al. Impact of Alzheimer disease patients' sleep disturbances on their caregivers. Geriatr Nurs 2018;39(1):60–5.
5. Ohayon MM, O'Hara R, Vitiello MV. Epidemiology of restless legs syndrome: a synthesis of the literature. Sleep Med Rev 2012;16(4):283–95.
6. Richards K, Shue VM, Beck CK, et al. Restless legs syndrome risk factors, behaviors, and diagnoses in persons with early to moderate dementia and sleep disturbance. Behav Sleep Med 2010;8(1):48–61.
7. Rose KM, Beck C, Tsai PF, et al. Sleep disturbances and nocturnal agitation behaviors in older adults with dementia. Sleep 2011;34(6):779–86.
8. Garcia-Borreguero D, Stillman P, Benes H, et al. Algorithms for the diagnosis and treatment of restless legs syndrome in primary care. BMC Neurol 2011;11(1):28.
9. Silber MH, Ehrenberg BL, Allen RP, et al. An algorithm for the management of restless legs syndrome. Mayo Clin Proc 2004;79(7):916–22.
10. Vignatelli L, Billiard M, Clarenbach P, et al. EFNS guidelines on management of restless legs syndrome and periodic limb movement disorder in sleep. Eur J Neurol 2006;13(10):1049–65.
11. Allen RP, Picchietti D, Hening WA, et al. Restless legs syndrome: diagnostic criteria, special considerations, and epidemiology. A report from the restless legs syndrome diagnosis and epidemiology workshop at the National Institutes of Health. Sleep Med 2003;4(2):101–19.
12. Hening WA. Current guidelines and standards of practice for restless legs syndrome. Am J Med 2007;120(suppl 1):S22–7.
13. Oertel WH, Trenkwalder C, Zucconi M, et al. State of the art in restless legs syndrome therapy: practice recommendations for treating restless legs syndrome. Mov Disord 2007;22(suppl 18):S466–75.
14. Trenkwalder C, Högl B, Winkelmann J. Recent advances in the diagnosis, genetics and treatment of restless legs syndrome. J Neurol 2009;256(4):539–53.
15. Boehm G, Wetter TC, Trenkwalder C. Periodic leg movements in RLS patients as compared to controls: are there differences beyond the PLM index? Sleep Med 2009;10(5):566–71.
16. Sforza E, Haba-Rubio J. Night-to-night variability in periodic leg movements in patients with restless legs syndrome. Sleep Med 2005;6(3):259–67.
17. Karroum EG, Golmard J-L, Leu-Semenescu S, et al. Sensations in restless legs syndrome. Sleep Med 2012;13(4):402–8.
18. Kerr S, McKinon W, Bentley A. Descriptors of restless legs syndrome sensations. Sleep Med 2012;13(4):409–13.
19. Whittom S, Dauvilliers Y, Pennestri MH, et al. Age-at-onset in restless legs syndrome: a clinical and polysomnographic study. Sleep Med 2007;9(1):54–9.
20. Allen RP, Bharmal M, Calloway M. Prevalence and disease burden of primary restless legs syndrome: results of a general population survey in the United States. Mov Disord 2011;26(1):114–20.
21. Phillips B, Hening W, Britz P, et al. Prevalence and correlates of restless legs syndrome: results from the 2005 National Sleep Foundation Poll. Chest 2006;129(1):76–80.
22. Earley CJ, Silber MH. Restless legs syndrome: understanding its consequences and the need for better treatment. Sleep Med 2010;11(9):807–15.

23. Allen RP, Picchietti DL, Garcia-Borreguero D, et al. Restless legs syndrome/Willis–Ekbom disease diagnostic criteria: updated International Restless Legs Syndrome Study Group (IRLSSG) consensus criteria—history, rationale, description, and significance. Sleep Med 2014;15(8):860–73.

24. Allen RP, Earley CJ. Restless legs syndrome: a review of clinical and pathophysiologic features. J Clin Neurophysiol 2001;18(2):128–47.

25. Trenkwalder C, Paulus W. Restless legs syndrome: pathophysiology, clinical presentation and management. Nat Rev Neurol 2010;6(6):337–46.

26. Allen R. Dopamine and iron in the pathophysiology of restless legs syndrome (RLS). Sleep Med 2004;5(4):385–91.

27. Belke M, Heverhagen JT, Keil B, et al. DTI and VBM reveal white matter changes without associated gray matter changes in patients with idiopathic restless legs syndrome. Brain Behav 2015;5(9):e00327.

28. Cuellar NG, Strumpf NE, Ratcliffe SJ. Symptoms of restless legs syndrome in older adults: outcomes on sleep quality, sleepiness, fatigue, depression, and quality of life. J Am Geriatr Soc 2007;55(9):1387–92.

29. Jean-Louis G, Magai CM, Cohen CI, et al. Ethnic differences in self-reported sleep problems in older adults. Sleep 2001;24(8):926–33.

30. Yeh P, Walters AS, Tsuang JW. Restless legs syndrome: a comprehensive overview on its epidemiology, risk factors, and treatment. Sleep Breath 2012;16(4):987–1007.

31. Berger K, Luedemann J, Trenkwalder C, et al. Sex and the risk of restless legs syndrome in the general population. Arch Intern Med 2004;164(2):196–202.

32. Allen RP, Auerbach S, Bahrain H, et al. The prevalence and impact of restless legs syndrome on patients with iron deficiency anemia. Am J Hematol 2013;88(4):261–4.

33. Trotti LM. Restless legs syndrome and sleep-related movement disorders. Continuum 2017;23(4):1005–16.

34. Bliwise DL, Zhang RH, Kutner NG. Medications associated with restless legs syndrome: a case-control study in the US Renal Data System (USRDS). Sleep Med 2014;15(10):1241–5.

35. Talarico G, Canevelli M, Tosto G, et al. Restless legs syndrome in a group of patients with Alzheimer's disease. Am J Alzheimers Dis Other Demen 2013;28(2):165–70.

36. Richards KC, Lichuan Y, Fry L. Sleep in long-term care settings. In: Kryger MH, Roth T, Dement WC, editors. Principles and practice in sleep medicine, 7th edition. New York: Elsiever, in press.

37. Ye L, Richards KC. Sleep and long-term care. Sleep Med Clin 2018;13(1):117–25.

38. Richards KC, Bost JE, Rogers VE, et al. Diagnostic accuracy of behavioral, activity, ferritin, and clinical indicators of restless legs syndrome. Sleep 2015;38(3):371–80.

39. Burbank F, Buchfuhrer M, Kopjar B, et al. Sleep improvement for restless legs syndrome patients. Part I: pooled analysis of two prospective, double-blind, sham-controlled, multi-center, randomized clinical studies of the effects of vibrating pads on RLS symptoms. J Parkinsonism Restless Legs Syndr 2013;2013:1–10.

40. Park A, Ambrogi K, Hade EM. Randomized pilot trial for the efficacy of the MMF07 foot massager and heat therapy for restless legs syndrome. PLoS One 2020;15(4):e0230951.

41. Lettieri CJ, Eliasson AH. Pneumatic compression devices are an effective therapy for restless legs syndrome: a prospective, randomized, double-blinded, sham-controlled trial. Chest 2009;135(1):74–80.

42. Aukerman MM, Aukerman D, Bayard M, et al. Exercise and restless legs syndrome: a randomized controlled trial. J Am Board Fam Med 2006;19(5):487–93.

43. Peters T, MacDonald R, Leach CMJ. Counterstrain manipulation in the treatment of restless legs syndrome: a pilot single-blind randomized controlled trial; the CARL trial. Int Musculoskelet Med 2012;34(4):136–40.

44. Innes KE, Selfe TK. The effects of a gentle yoga program on sleep, mood, and blood pressure in older women with restless legs syndrome (RLS): a preliminary randomized controlled trial. Evid Based Complement Alternat Med 2012;2012: 294058.

45. Happe S, Evers S, Thiedemann C, et al. Whole body and local cryotherapy in restless legs syndrome: a randomized, single-blind, controlled parallel group pilot study. J Neurol Sci 2016;370:7–12.

46. Garcia-Borreguero D, Silber MH, Winkelman JW, et al. Guidelines for the first-line treatment of restless legs syndrome/Willis–Ekbom disease, prevention and treatment of dopaminergic augmentation: a combined task force of the IRLSSG, EURLSSG, and the RLS-foundation. Sleep Med 2016;21:1–11.

47. Gonzalez-Latapi P, Malkani R. Update on restless legs syndrome: from mechanisms to treatment. Curr Neurol Neurosci Rep 2019;19(8):54.

48. Cortese S, Konofal E, Lecendreux M, et al. Restless legs syndrome and attention-deficit/hyperactivity disorder: a review of the literature. Sleep 2005;28(8): 1007–13.

Sleep after Traumatic Brain Injury

Kris B. Weymann, PhD, RN[a,b,]*, Jennifer M. Rourke, MS, RN, AGCNS-BC, CCRN[c]

KEYWORDS

- Traumatic brain injury • Sleep • Sleep–wake disorders • Insomnia • Fatigue

KEY POINTS

- Sleep disturbances are common after traumatic brain injury of all levels of severity, and can arise early after injury and persist for years.
- Sleep disturbances interfere with functional recovery from traumatic brain injury.
- Preventing, recognizing, and addressing impaired sleep in the in-patient setting can promote recovery.
- Early and ongoing education about the importance of sleep and sleep hygiene strategies should be included in care to improve recovery from traumatic brain injury.

INTRODUCTION

Sleep is essential for function.[1] Some specific functions of sleep, such as memory consolidation and learning, have been demonstrated.[2,3] Yet overall functions of sleep remain poorly understood. Four of 6 viable theories of sleep function reviewed by Krueger and colleagues[4] focus on brain health—promoting neural connectivity, restoring neural networks to maintain cognitive and behavioral performance, allowing for the flushing of substances from the brain tissue, and restoring brain energy stores. The role of sleep in brain recovery from traumatic brain injury (TBI) may be important, but it is not understood. TBI is defined as altered brain function from an external force, rated as mild—such as concussion—or moderate or severe, usually determined by score on the Glasgow Coma Scale. Although each TBI is unique, there are some common problems that arise from this heterogeneous disorder.

Sleep problems are among the most common complaints after TBI of all levels of severity, and these problems can persist for years after injury.[5–10] A meta-analysis of 21 studies found that about 50% (95% confidence interval, 49%–51%) of people had sleep disturbances after a TBI.[11] In a prospective study of predominantly male

[a] VA Portland Health Care System, Portland, OR, USA; [b] Oregon Health & Science University, School of Nursing, SN-6S, 3455 Southwest US Veterans Hospital Road, Portland, OR 97239, USA; [c] VA Portland Health Care System, P2IESD, 3710 Southwest US Veterans Hospital Road, Portland, OR 97239, USA
* Corresponding author. Oregon Health & Science University, School of Nursing, SN-6S, 3455 Southwest US Veterans Hospital Road, Portland, OR 97239.
E-mail address: weymannk@ohsu.edu

Nurs Clin N Am 56 (2021) 275–286
https://doi.org/10.1016/j.cnur.2021.02.006
0029-6465/21/Published by Elsevier Inc.

nursing.theclinics.com

participants with a TBI, 72% and 67% had a sleep–wake disturbance 6 months and 3 years after injury, respectively.[10] Among veterans, 56% of 527 participants reported clinically significant poor sleep persisting for an average of 6 years, independent of a variety of factors that could impair sleep.[9] With 2.8 million emergency room visits in 2013 in the United States for TBI,[12] and evidence of increasing rates of injury,[13] understanding how to improve recovery from a TBI is critical. Preventing, recognizing, and addressing sleep disorders after a TBI can contribute to promoting functional recovery. The evidence of sleep importance after a TBI, along with clinical features and management of the most common sleep disorders after a TBI in adults are presented in this article.

IMPORTANCE OF SLEEP IN RECOVERY FROM TRAUMATIC BRAIN INJURY

There is increasing evidence indicating the importance of sleep for recovery from a TBI (**Fig. 1**).[14] In a study of 238 individuals evaluated within 24 hours after a TBI, those with trouble falling asleep or with short sleep were more functionally impaired during the first 6 months after injury than those with good sleep.[15] In a study of 64 participants, those with sleep features within the first 14 days after a TBI as determined by electroencephalography were found to have earlier participation in rehabilitative therapies and better functional recovery, independent of Glasgow Coma Scale scores at admission.[16] Disrupted sleep was found to predict agitation after a moderate to severe brain

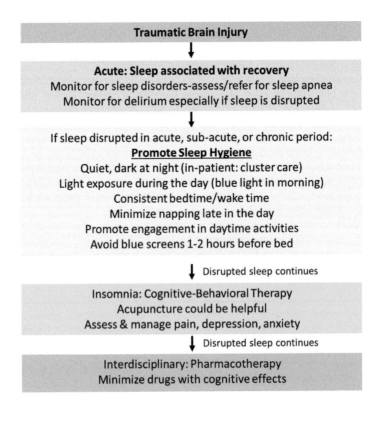

Fig. 1. Restoring sleep after traumatic brain injury.[54–56]

injury,[17] a concern given the risk of delirium in patients with a TBI.[18] In a prospective study, poor sleep in the intensive care unit increased the chance of developing delirium by 10.7 times.[19] In a study of 30 people in the acute phase of a moderate or severe TBI, the reappearance of a normal sleep–wake cycle, measured with wrist actigraphy, was found to be synchronous with the ability to follow commands with appropriate verbal and motor responses. The authors suggested that a common underlying brain mechanism may support both sleep–wake cycle and cognitive function.[20]

The association of sleep with function and recovery was found to continue into the rehabilitative period. Starting at admission to rehabilitation after a moderate to severe TBI, sleep–wake cycle disturbance and weekly scores on the Cognitive Test for Delirium were significantly associated, indicating that those with sleep–wake cycle disturbance had greater cognitive impairment when matched for demographic and injury variables.[21] In a study of 59 patients with TBI recruited from a rehabilitation unit, disrupted sleep measured both objectively and subjectively was associated with poorer motor outcomes and a slower recovery.[22]

An association of sleep with function and recovery was found up to 2 years after injury. In a study of 92 workers after an average of about 6 months after a mild TBI (mTBI), insomnia was the only significant covariate in a fully adjusted work disability model. The authors concluded the importance of diagnosis and management of insomnia in persons with a mTBI to support higher function among workers.[23] Comparing those with a mTBI with persistent sleep disturbances with those whose sleep disturbances had resolved after injury, persistent sleep disturbance at 6 months after injury, independent of psychological distress, predicted a poorer outcome.[24] At 18 months after injury, Imbach and colleagues[25] found that those with a TBI needed an additional hour of sleep compared with matched controls, and 67% of those with TBI had chronic objective excessive daytime sleepiness compared with 19% of controls. Patients under-reported sleep need and excessive daytime sleepiness. The authors concluded that untreated sleep–wake disorders in those with a TBI could impair quality of life and risk safety.[25] At 5 years after TBI, there was a 1.36-fold increase in sleep disturbance compared with non-TBI controls in a population-based cohort study including 6932 with TBI and 34,660 matched controls.[8]

It is not known why sleep is so commonly disrupted after TBI. A variety of mechanisms have been proposed, including neurotransmitter disruption to or from the hypothalamus, brain stem, or pineal gland. This disruption could affect glutamate, galanin, or melatonin signaling involved with sleep, and/or disruption of neurotransmitters affecting wakefulness—including orexin, histamine, serotonin, dopamine, norepinephrine, and other substancess.[7] Some mechanisms have been elucidated by studies in animal models, with more research after a TBI needed.[5] Even without clear diagnostic tools, recognizing and intervening to restore sleep after a TBI is an important health and safety issue.

SLEEP CONCERNS IN ACUTE PERIOD AFTER TRAUMATIC BRAIN INJURY

An ongoing concern for patients hospitalized after a TBI is the overlap of risk factors and presentation of impaired sleep and the bidirectional relationship with delirium, particularly the hypoactive subtype characterized by lethargy and sedation.[26] One-half of patients with a mild to moderate TBI developed delirium within the first 4 days after injury, with 69.4% developing delirium during the hospitalization.[18]

The initial treatment of sleep–wake disorders after a TBI should include nonpharmacologic interventions to modify environmental and behavioral factors (**Table 1**).[27] In a

Table 1
Clinics care points

Clinical Care Points to Promote Sleep in the Hospital	
Daytime	**Nighttime**
• Lights on during the day. • Position near a window if possible. • Promote patient engagement—visitors, hearing aids, and eye glasses as indicated. • Reorient the patient, provide clock. • Minimize late afternoon naps. • Eat meals at regular times. • Exercise/progressive mobility. • Limit evening caffeine.	• Minimize light in the evening and during the night. • Limit blue screen time in the evening. • Limit noise; consider white noise. • Provide a sleep mask/ear plugs if not contraindicated. • Encourage a consistent bedtime routine. • Bundle tasks. • Complete procedures at the beginning or the end of the shift.

review of sleep disruptions in the intensive care unit, 21% of disruptions were from sound, with patient care activities, illness severity, and pain also associated with sleep disruption.[26]

The success of nonpharmacologic interventions may be limited when there is impaired cognition.[26] A multifaceted and multidisciplinary approach including medication for sleep–wake disorders can improve patient outcomes by decreasing daytime sleepiness, neurobehavioral impairments, and the risk of delirium.[27,28] In a randomized, controlled, double-blinded study, daytime alertness improved in patients with a mild to severe TBI after an evening dose of melatonin.[29] Additional medications for sleep–wake disorders may include antidepressants; GABA agonists such as zolpidem; alpha-1 receptor adrenergic blockers such as prazosin, which can be beneficial when post-traumatic stress disorder is associated with a TBI; and careful use of benzodiazepines. Anticholinergic medication for sleep–wake disorders in a patient with a TBI should be avoided for the first 3 months owing to adverse cognitive effects.[29]

COMMON SLEEP–WAKE DISTURBANCES AFTER TRAUMATIC BRAIN INJURY: SUBACUTE AND CHRONIC PERIODS

Common sleep–wake disorders after TBI include hypersomnia, insomnia, sleep–wake cycle disturbance, sleep apnea, excessive daytime sleepiness, and fatigue.[6,11] These disorders can overlap and likely contribute to excessive daytime sleepiness and fatigue as symptoms of a sleep disorder.[30] The frequency of occurrence in the subacute and chronic periods; the clinical features are presented in **Table 2**.

Hypersomnia

Hypersomnia, or pleiosomnia, is an increased need to sleep, over a 24-hour period, as compared with before the injury. Unrelieved pain after a mTBI was found to be associated with a greater number of naps during the day at 1 month after injury.[31] It should be taken into account that the recommended amount of sleep for a healthy adult is 7 to 9 hours,[32] which may not be reflected in the baseline sleep, because those with short sleep are at increased risk of injury.[33] Hypersomnia often manifests as sleep need during the day, making it difficult to distinguish from excessive daytime sleepiness, which is discussed separately.

Insomnia

Insomnia is delayed sleep onset, awakenings with difficulty returning to sleep, and/or waking too early, resulting in distress and daytime subjective impairment. Insomnia

Table 2
Common sleep disorders after traumatic brain injury and frequency in subacute and chronic time frames

Sleep Disorder	Frequency	Clinical Features
Increased sleep need (hypersomnia/ pleiosomnia)	22%–49%	Increased sleep need of 2 h over 24 h as compared with before injury. Other causes of increased sleep need excluded.
Insomnia	29%–65%	Difficulty falling asleep or staying asleep, resulting in distress and daytime subjective impairment. Consider possible circadian rhythm disorder.
Sleep–wake cycle (circadian rhythm) disturbance	36%–84%	Sleeping during the day and awake at night, or lacking a clear pattern of sleep and wake, or a delayed sleep pattern
Sleep apnea	25%–49%	Cessation or reduction of breathing while asleep. May be preexisting.
Excessive daytime sleepiness	42%–47%	Decreased alertness or drowsiness during the day; possible unintentional sleep at inappropriate times.
Fatigue	>60%	Subjective feeling of tiredness not proportional to recent activity and interfering with usual function.

can be assessed with the Insomnia Severity Index, a 7-item measure with a total score of 28 points, with a score of 15 or more indicating clinical insomnia.[34] Insomnia is a common problem after a TBI, with a frequency of 33% to 65% in the subacute and chronic time periods,[35,36] and can result in decreased satisfaction in life, increased disability upon return to work, anxiety, and depression.[35] Insomnia can contribute to excessive daytime sleepiness and symptoms of fatigue. In a sample of 334 patients, those with insomnia after a TBI were found to have worse sleep hygiene, supporting that strategy as an intervention.[35] Insomnia can mask a circadian rhythm disorder, which necessitates detection and treatment to support recovery.[37]

Sleep–Wake Cycle Disturbance and Circadian Rhythm Disturbance

A sleep–wake cycle disturbance can manifest as lacking a clear pattern of sleep and wake, or being awake at night and sleeping during the day. It can also manifest as a delayed sleep phase that can be overlooked and interpreted as insomnia,[37] or as an advanced sleep phase.[38] The management of a sleep–wake cycle disturbance is similar with and without a TBI, although prolonged hospitalization, poor light exposure, sedative effects of medications, and decreased mobility increase the difficulty of management after TBI.[38] Morning light therapy to treat delayed sleep phase and evening light therapy to treat advanced sleep phase have been demonstrated to be effective,[38] keeping in mind that individuals with a TBI frequently have increased sensitivity to light.[39] Exciting recent findings indicate improved retinohypothalamic function after blue light therapy after a TBI, suggesting that addressing any sleep–wake cycle disturbance may have additional benefits in brain recovery.[40]

The frequency of sleep–wake cycle disturbance after a TBI ranges from 36%[41] to 84% at admission to rehabilitation, and decreasing to 66% at 1 month after the injury.[42] The presence of moderate to severe sleep–wake cycle disturbance predicated the duration of rehabilitation hospital length stay.[42] Interventions to restore night sleep in the hospital setting are important because disrupted sleep is associated with delirium, which is common after a TBI.[18] Supporting sleep hygiene and addressing pain or discomfort that could interfere with sleep are important early interventions to both prevent and address sleep–wake cycle disturbances.

Sleep Apnea and Sleep-Disordered Breathing

Sleep apnea is cessation or inadequate breathing while asleep. It might be newly occurring after a TBI, or may be preexisting, and can arise from partial or complete obstruction of the upper airway or a central cause. Both obstructive sleep apnea (OSA) and central apnea are more prevalent in those with a TBI[33] and may result from brain injury, decreased arousal, impaired respiratory function, and surrounding tissue pressure. If preexisting and not adequately treated, the excessive daytime sleepiness or fatigue that results from poor sleep may be associated with the occurrence of the TBI, such as a motor vehicle crash or other injury resulting from decreased alertness.[33]

Apneic or hypopneic events during sleep lead to decreased oxygenation and subsequent activation of the sympathetic nervous system. Sympathetic nervous system activation results in arousal and taking a needed breath, often without waking. It also results in increased pulse and blood pressure, increased blood sugar, and increased inflammatory signaling, which can increase cardiovascular risks and disease. The assessment of risk of OSA can include the STOP-BANG assessment tool, which has 8 yes or no questions on snoring, being tired, observed apnea, high blood pressure, a body mass index of more than 35 kg/m^2, age older than 50 years, neck circumference 16 inches or larger, and male gender. An answer of yes on 5 of the 8 questions indicates high risk of OSA.[43,44] An overnight sleep test determines a diagnosis of OSA. A core component of treatment of OSA is positive airway pressure (PAP) therapy, where pressurized air stenting open the airway prevents airway collapse. Although the side effects of PAP therapy are minimal, adherence to PAP therapy after a TBI can be low. This finding indicates an increased importance in education of those with sleep apnea about the importance of adequate treatment.[45,46] Educational, behavioral, troubleshooting, and telemonitoring interventions were found in a meta-analysis to significantly improve PAP adherence.[47]

Excessive Daytime Sleepiness

Excessive daytime sleepiness is the inability to remain alert during the day, perhaps with unintentional sleep at inappropriate times, such as falling asleep when in a conversation or while driving. It can be a component of hypersomnia, but with the difference of a daytime focus and an intention to be awake. It is often associated with other sleep disorders that result in poor sleep at night and disrupted wake during the day. Using the criteria of a mean sleep latency of less than 10 minutes on the Multiple Sleep Latency Test, 1 study with 71 participants in a rehabilitation center after TBI reported that 47% had excessive daytime sleepiness. Participants with excessive daytime sleepiness did not rate themselves with this disorder. In addition, there was no association of sleep disorders with psychopathology, including dysthymic disorder, major depression, or anxiety in this selected cohort.[48] Although people with excessive daytime sleepiness might have an underlying sleep disorder, these participants had overnight sleep evaluation for sleep apnea and other sleep disorders. OSA was diagnosed in 4 patients, and probable narcolepsy in 1 patient, leaving 28 (39%) with excessive daytime sleepiness with no likely underlying cause other than the TBI. In a study of 118 participants in rehabilitation 6 to 8 weeks after injury, excessive daytime sleepiness determined by the Epworth Sleepiness Scale[49] score of 10 or greater was found in 41.7%. Anxiety was associated with excessive daytime sleepiness in a multivariate analysis. The authors concluded that anxiety should be assessed and treated to improve sleep outcomes in this population.[50] Both studies found rates of excessive daytime sleepiness after a TBI higher than the rate of 9% to 28% in the general population.[51]

Fatigue

Fatigue is one of the most common symptoms after a TBI, often persisting for years.[35] Fatigue, which is multidimensional, has been defined as a "distressing, persistent, subjective sense of physical, emotional, and/or cognitive tiredness or exhaustion… that is, not proportional to recent activity and interferes with usual functioning."[52] Fatigue can result from disrupted sleep from any cause. Fatigue after a brain injury can be related to increased cognitive or motor effort, depending on the location of brain injury, rather than, or in addition to, impaired sleep. Those with fatigue after a TBI had greater daytime sleepiness, worse sleep hygiene, more profound disability, and lower satisfaction with life.[35] In a large cohort of community-based patients with a TBI, fatigue after a TBI was not related to injury severity, age, orthopedic injury, or employment status. Fatigue after a TBI was moderately associated with pain, taking analgesic medication, female sex, depression, anxiety, and greater time after the injury. In addition, impaired attention and information processing speed were also associated with increased fatigue in those with TBI as compared with healthy controls.[53]

INTERVENTIONS TO PROMOTE RECOVERY

Interventions to improve sleep after TBI improves recovery.[54–56] Sleep apnea suspected after TBI needs to be addressed, which is discussed in the section on Sleep Apnea. In the acute period of TBI, bidirectional relationships between sleep and agitation, post-traumatic confusion, and cognitive impairment seem to exist, and improving sleep may help resolve these other symptoms during early recovery from a TBI.[57]

Interventions for sleep after a TBI have been tested in some studies that did not separate the different sleep disorders. In an inpatient rehabilitation setting, sleep hygiene including 30 minutes of blue light in the morning, restricted caffeine after noon, naps limited to 30 minutes during the day, lights out at an agreed upon time based on pre-TBI preferences, and a restriction of centrally acting medications were together found to significantly improve actigraph sleep metrics.[54] Morning blue light is known to advance sleep phase, which can restore circadian rhythm in someone with a phase delay, which can occur after a TBI.[38] In a review of interventions to address sleep problems after TBI, sleep hygiene education, cognitive behavioral therapy for insomnia, morning blue light therapy, problem solving treatment, and prazosin were evaluated to be beneficial to improve sleep. There was mixed evidence in this review supporting exercise interventions.[55] Cognitive behavioral therapy for insomnia has also been shown to be effective with Internet delivery, increasing the availability of this intervention for treating insomnia.[58]

After a TBI occurring at least 3 months earlier, a randomized control trial of high-intensity blue light therapy for 45 minutes each morning for 4 weeks decreased fatigue and daytime sleepiness during the treatment period with evidence of a trend toward preinjury levels 4 weeks after treatment cessation. These improvements were not found in control groups (10 participants per group) receiving lower intensity yellow light therapy or no treatment.[59]

The effects of morning blue light exposure, versus amber light exposure, was tested in a randomized control trial of 32 adults with a mTBI within the previous 18 months, but at least 4 weeks after injury. After 6 weeks of light exposure, those in the blue light group had phase-advanced sleep timing, decreased daytime sleepiness, and improved executive functioning. Participants in the blue light group also had an increased volume of the brain posterior thalamus, increased thalamocortical functional connectivity, and increased axonal integrity in these pathways. The authors concluded that interventions targeting the retinohypothalamic system could improve recovery from brain injury.[40]

Some studies reported benefits of modafinil in treating fatigue or excessive daytime sleepiness, but a meta-analysis of modafinil reported inconsistent results in the small studies.[60]

Assessing and treating anxiety, depression, and pain could help with improving sleep and/or managing fatigue. Assessing cognitive impairment, and assistance with tools to measure or limit cognitive burden, could also help with managing fatigue after a TBI, because sensory overstimulation after a brain injury can be interpreted as fatigue.[61] In a pilot study of 24 participants to compare the efficacy of acupuncture with medication in treating insomnia up to 5 years after a TBI, the authors reported that acupuncture had a beneficial effect, improving cognition and the perception of sleep quality even without a difference in sleep time between the acupuncture and medication groups. Because acupuncture has been reported to decrease insomnia after a stroke and in other neurologic disorders, the authors concluded that a larger study is warranted in those with a TBI.[62]

DISCUSSION AND SUMMARY

Sleep disturbances are common after a TBI and interfere with recovery. Some of the sleep disorders, such as OSA, have known, effective therapies, although educational and behavioral interventions are warranted to ensure adherence to prescribed PAP therapy to treat OSA after a TBI.[45,46] Taking the other sleep disorders together, because there can be quite a bit of overlap, sleep hygiene interventions, including morning blue light, restricted caffeine, time-limited daytime naps, limited use of blue light screens in the evening before bed, and a consistent bed time with lights out, were well-tolerated and improved sleep in inpatient rehabilitation and community settings.[54,55]

There is increasing evidence supporting the use of morning blue light to address sleep problems after a mTBI during rehabilitation between 1 and 18 months after injury. However, a high-intensity light might not be appropriate in the acute care setting within the first month after TBI owing to increased sensory sensitivity.[39] General sleep hygiene practices that include at least 30 minutes of morning exposure to sunlight through a window may improve sleep in the hospital setting if the clinical condition allows.[63]

Participants with a TBI were found to have increased sleep 18 months after injury, suggesting either a possible benefit of sleep in long-term recovery or persistent sleep impairment.[25] Sleep hygiene is a safe, well-tolerated, low-cost, effective approach to improving sleep in a variety of populations. Early and ongoing education about managing symptoms after a TBI, including sleep hygiene, can improve rehabilitation and recovery.[64] Systematic approaches and development of evidence-based educational interventions supporting long-term recovery after a TBI are needed.[64]

DISCLOSURE

The authors have nothing to disclose. The contents do not represent the views of the U.S. Department of Veterans Affairs or the United States Government.

REFERENCES

1. Krause AJ, Simon EB, Mander BA, et al. The sleep-deprived human brain. Nat Rev Neurosci 2017;18(7):404–18.
2. Boyce R, Glasgow SD, Williams S, et al. Causal evidence for the role of REM sleep theta rhythm in contextual memory consolidation. Science 2016; 352(6287):812–6.
3. Diekelmann S, Born J. The memory function of sleep. Nat Rev Neurosci 2010; 11(2):114–26.
4. Krueger JM, Frank MG, Wisor JP, et al. Sleep function: toward elucidating an enigma. Sleep Med Rev 2016;28:46–54.
5. Sandsmark DK, Elliott JE, Lim MM. Sleep-wake disturbances after traumatic brain injury: synthesis of human and animal studies. Sleep 2017;40(5):zsx044.
6. Ouellet MC, Beaulieu-Bonneau S, Morin CM. Sleep-wake disturbances after traumatic brain injury. Lancet Neurol 2015;14(7):746–57.
7. Wickwire EM, Williams SG, Roth T, et al. Sleep, sleep disorders, and mild traumatic brain injury. what we know and what we need to know: findings from a National Working Group. Neurotherapeutics 2016;13(2):403–17.
8. Wang YJ, Chang WC, Wu CC, et al. Increased short- and long-term risk of sleep disorders in people with traumatic brain injury. Neuropsychol Rehabil 2021;31(2): 211–30.
9. Martindale SL, Farrell-Carnahan LV, Ulmer CS, et al. Sleep quality in returning veterans: the influence of mild traumatic brain injury. Rehabil Psychol 2017;62(4): 563–70.
10. Kempf J, Werth E, Kaiser PR, et al. Sleep-wake disturbances 3 years after traumatic brain injury. J Neurol Neurosurg Psychiatr 2010;81(12):1402–5.
11. Mathias JL, Alvaro PK. Prevalence of sleep disturbances, disorders, and problems following traumatic brain injury: a meta-analysis. Sleep Med 2012;13(7): 898–905.
12. Taylor CA, Bell JM, Breiding MJ, et al. Traumatic brain injury-related emergency department visits, hospitalizations, and deaths - United States, 2007 and 2013. MMWR Surveill Summ 2017;66(9):1–16.
13. Peterson AB, Kegler SR. Deaths from fall-related traumatic brain injury - United States, 2008-2017. MMWR Morb Mortal Wkly Rep 2020;69(9):225–30.
14. Lowe A, Neligan A, Greenwood R. Sleep disturbance and recovery during rehabilitation after traumatic brain injury: a systematic review. Disabil Rehabil 2020; 42(8):1041–54.
15. Kalmbach DA, Conroy DA, Falk H, et al. Poor sleep is linked to impeded recovery from traumatic brain injury. Sleep 2018;41(10):zsy147.
16. Sandsmark DK, Kumar MA, Woodward CS, et al. Sleep features on continuous electroencephalography predict rehabilitation outcomes after severe traumatic brain injury. J Head Trauma Rehabil 2016;31(2):101–7.
17. Draganich C, Gerber D, Monden KR, et al. Disrupted sleep predicts next day agitation following moderate to severe brain injury. Brain Inj 2019;33(9):1194–9.
18. Maneewong J, Maneeton B, Maneeton N, et al. Delirium after a traumatic brain injury: predictors and symptom patterns. Neuropsychiatr Dis Treat 2017;13: 459–65.
19. Li X, Zhang L, Gong F, et al. Incidence and risk factors for delirium in older patients following intensive care unit admission: a prospective observational study. J Nurs Res 2020;28(4):e101.

20. Duclos C, Dumont M, Arbour C, et al. Parallel recovery of consciousness and sleep in acute traumatic brain injury. Neurology 2017;88(3):268.

21. Holcomb EM, Towns S, Kamper JE, et al. The relationship between sleep-wake cycle disturbance and trajectory of cognitive recovery during acute traumatic brain injury. J Head Trauma Rehabil 2016;31(2):108–16.

22. Fleming MK, Smejka T, Henderson Slater D, et al. Sleep disruption after brain injury is associated with worse motor outcomes and slower functional recovery. Neurorehabil Neural Repair 2020;34(7):661–71.

23. Mollayeva T, Pratt B, Mollayeva S, et al. The relationship between insomnia and disability in workers with mild traumatic brain injury/concussion: insomnia and disability in chronic mild traumatic brain injury. Sleep Med 2016;20:157–66.

24. Chan LG, Feinstein A. Persistent sleep disturbances independently predict poorer functional and social outcomes 1 year after mild traumatic brain injury. J Head Trauma Rehabil 2015;30(6):E67–75.

25. Imbach LL, Büchele F, Valko PO, et al. Sleep–wake disorders persist 18 months after traumatic brain injury but remain underrecognized. Neurology 2016;86(21):1945.

26. Chang VA, Owens RL, LaBuzetta JN. Impact of sleep deprivation in the neurological intensive care unit: a narrative review. Neurocrit Care 2020;32(2):596–608.

27. Grimm J. Sleep deprivation in the intensive care patient. Crit Care Nurse 2020;40(2):e16–24.

28. Driver S, Stork R. Pharmacological management of sleep after traumatic brain injury. NeuroRehabilitation 2018;43(3):347–53.

29. Bhatnagar S, Iaccarino MA, Zafonte R. Pharmacotherapy in rehabilitation of post-acute traumatic brain injury. Brain Res 2016;1640(Pt A):164–79.

30. Monderer R, Ahmed IM, Thorpy M. Evaluation of the sleepy patient: differential diagnosis. Sleep Med Clin 2020;15(2):155–66.

31. Suzuki Y, Khoury S, El-Khatib H, et al. Individuals with pain need more sleep in the early stage of mild traumatic brain injury. Sleep Med 2017;33:36–42.

32. Watson NF, Badr MS, Belenky G, et al. Joint Consensus Statement of the American Academy of Sleep Medicine and sleep research society on the recommended amount of sleep for a healthy adult: methodology and discussion. Sleep 2015;38(8):1161–83.

33. Holcomb EM, Schwartz DJ, McCarthy M, et al. Incidence, characterization, and predictors of sleep apnea in consecutive brain injury rehabilitation admissions. J Head Trauma Rehabil 2016;31(2):82–100.

34. Bastien CH, Vallières A, Morin CM. Validation of the Insomnia Severity Index as an outcome measure for insomnia research. Sleep Med 2001;2(4):297–307.

35. Cantor JB, Bushnik T, Cicerone K, et al. Insomnia, fatigue, and sleepiness in the first 2 years after traumatic brain injury: an NIDRR TBI model system module study. J Head Trauma Rehabil 2012;27(6):E1–14.

36. Zhou Y, Greenwald BD. Update on insomnia after mild traumatic brain injury. Brain Sci 2018;8(12):223.

37. Zalai DM, Girard TA, Cusimano MD, et al. Circadian rhythm in the assessment of postconcussion insomnia: a cross-sectional observational study. CMAJ Open 2020;8(1):e142–7.

38. Aoun R, Rawal H, Attarian H, et al. Impact of traumatic brain injury on sleep: an overview. Nat Sci Sleep 2019;11:131–40.

39. Elliott JE, Opel RA, Weymann KB, et al. Sleep disturbances in traumatic brain injury: associations with sensory sensitivity. J Clin Sleep Med 2018;14(7):1177–86.

40. Killgore WDS, Vanuk JR, Shane BR, et al. A randomized, double-blind, placebo-controlled trial of blue wavelength light exposure on sleep and recovery of brain structure, function, and cognition following mild traumatic brain injury. Neurobiol Dis 2020;134:104679.

41. Ayalon L, Borodkin K, Dishon L, et al. Circadian rhythm sleep disorders following mild traumatic brain injury. Neurology 2007;68(14):1136–40.

42. Nakase-Richardson R, Sherer M, Barnett SD, et al. Prospective evaluation of the nature, course, and impact of acute sleep abnormality after traumatic brain injury. Arch Phys Med Rehabil 2013;94(5):875–82.

43. Chung F, Abdullah HR, Liao P. STOP-bang questionnaire: a practical approach to screen for obstructive sleep apnea. Chest 2016;149(3):631–8.

44. Chung F, Yegneswaran B, Liao P, et al. STOP questionnaire: a tool to screen patients for obstructive sleep apnea. Anesthesiology 2008;108(5):812–21.

45. Collen JF, Lettieri CJ, Hoffman M. The impact of posttraumatic stress disorder on CPAP adherence in patients with obstructive sleep apnea. J Clin Sleep Med 2012;8(6):667–72.

46. Lettieri CJ, Williams SG, Collen JF, et al. Treatment of obstructive sleep apnea: achieving adherence to positive airway pressure treatment and dealing with complications. Sleep Med Clin 2020;15(2):227–40.

47. Patil SP, Ayappa IA, Caples SM, et al. Treatment of adult obstructive sleep apnea with positive airway pressure: an American Academy of Sleep Medicine systematic review, meta-analysis, and GRADE assessment. J Clin Sleep Med 2019; 15(2):301–34.

48. Masel BE, Scheibel RS, Kimbark T, et al. Excessive daytime sleepiness in adults with brain injuries. Arch Phys Med Rehabil 2001;82(11):1526–32.

49. Johns MW. A new method for measuring daytime sleepiness: the Epworth sleepiness scale. Sleep 1991;14(6):540–5.

50. Crichton T, Singh R, Abosi-Appeadu K, et al. Excessive daytime sleepiness after traumatic brain injury. Brain Inj 2020;34(11):1525–31.

51. Jaussent I, Morin CM, Ivers H, et al. Incidence, worsening and risk factors of daytime sleepiness in a population-based 5-year longitudinal study. Sci Rep 2017; 7(1):1372.

52. Bower JE. Cancer-related fatigue–mechanisms, risk factors, and treatments. Nat Rev Clin Oncol 2014;11(10):597–609.

53. Ponsford JL, Ziino C, Parcell DL, et al. Fatigue and sleep disturbance following traumatic brain injury–their nature, causes, and potential treatments. J Head Trauma Rehabil 2012;27(3):224–33.

54. Makley MJ, Gerber D, Newman JK, et al. Optimized Sleep After Brain Injury (OSABI): a pilot study of a sleep hygiene intervention for individuals with moderate to severe traumatic brain injury. Neurorehabil Neural Repair 2020;34(2): 111–21.

55. Bogdanov S, Naismith S, Lah S. Sleep outcomes following sleep-hygiene-related interventions for individuals with traumatic brain injury: a systematic review. Brain Inj 2017;31(4):422–33.

56. Jaffe M. Sleep & traumatic brain injury. Pract Neurol 2019. Available at: http://v2.practicalneurology.com/2019/04/sleep–traumatic-brain-injury/.

57. Poulsen I, Langhorn L, Egerod I, et al. Sleep and agitation during subacute traumatic brain injury rehabilitation: a scoping review. Aust Crit Care 2021;34(1): 76–82.

58. van der Zweerde T, Lancee J, Ida Luik A, et al. Internet-delivered cognitive behavioral therapy for insomnia: tailoring cognitive behavioral therapy for insomnia for patients with chronic insomnia. Sleep Med Clin 2020;15(2):117–31.

59. Sinclair KL, Ponsford JL, Taffe J, et al. Randomized controlled trial of light therapy for fatigue following traumatic brain injury. Neurorehabil Neural Repair 2014; 28(4):303–13.

60. Sheng P, Hou L, Wang X, et al. Efficacy of modafinil on fatigue and excessive day-time sleepiness associated with neurological disorders: a systematic review and meta-analysis. PLoS One 2013;8(12):e81802.

61. Juengst SB, Nabasny A, Terhorst L. Neurobehavioral symptoms in community-dwelling adults with and without chronic traumatic brain injury: differences by age, gender, education, and health condition. Front Neurol 2019;10:1210.

62. Zollman FS, Larson EB, Wasek-Throm LK, et al. Acupuncture for treatment of insomnia in patients with traumatic brain injury: a pilot intervention study. J Head Trauma Rehabil 2012;27(2):135–42.

63. Shimura A, Sugiura K, Inoue M, et al. Which sleep hygiene factors are important? comprehensive assessment of lifestyle habits and job environment on sleep among office workers. Sleep Health 2020;6(3):288–98.

64. Hart T, Driver S, Sander A, et al. Traumatic brain injury education for adult patients and families: a scoping review. Brain Inj 2018;32(11):1295–306.

Sleep and Physiological Function

Sleep, Aging, and Daily Functioning

Amy S. Berkley, PhD, RN

KEYWORDS

- Older adults • Sleep • Sleep disorders • Daily functioning • Insomnia
- Sleep assessment

KEY POINTS

- Disrupted or poor quality sleep is not a part of normal aging.
- Older and younger adults require the same 7 to 9 hours of healthy sleep.
- Questions about sleep and sleep quality should be included in any patient interview.

INTRODUCTION

Good sleep is vital to physical and mental health. People who do not sleep well or do not sleep enough face fatigue, impaired cognition, and a host of metabolic problems leading to diabetes and obesity, as well as a decreased quality of life.[1] However, for older adults, the issue is more serious. Older adults who do not sleep well at night frequently have difficulty sustaining attention in the daytime, display slower physical response times, and have memory issues, which may contribute to depression or early dementia.[2,3] Poor nighttime sleep can also lead to daytime napping, which can increase disorientation and social isolation in older adults.[4,5] The Institute of Medicine has declared sleep disorders and sleep deprivation "an unmet public health problem" for the whole population while noting that for older adults the problem is too often overlooked.[6] This article provides an overview of the ways sleep changes as we age, and the current diagnosis and treatment recommendations for the most common sleep disorders faced by older adults, supported by nursing case studies. It concludes with a review of novel interventions for sleep promotion, and future directions for clinical practice and sleep research.

SLEEP IN NORMAL AGING

Despite common perceptions that sleep difficulties are a part of normal aging, many older adults sleep well and report few sleep issues. However, there are recognized

The author has nothing to disclose.
The author(s) received no financial support for the research, authorship, and/or publication of this article.
University of Kansas School of Nursing, Mail Stop 2029, 3901 Rainbow Boulevard, Kansas City, KS 66160, USA
E-mail address: aberkley3@kumc.edu

physiologic changes that are associated with changes to sleep. Sleep duration and quality vary across the human lifespan and standards of "normative" sleep are affected by environments, societal roles, cultural patterns, and living arrangements, as well as by physiologic changes associated with advancing age.[7,8] Contrary to popular beliefs about aging, research has shown that healthy older adults and younger adults require comparable amounts of sleep, but that multiple health, social, and environmental risk factors make achieving that need much more difficult as people age.[9,10]

Older adults' sleep has been described as more "fragile,"[10] more "easily disrupted,"[11] and "more disjointed"[12] than that of younger adults. How much of this fragility or disjointedness is due to external, potentially modifiable factors such as stress, pharmacology, pain, nocturia, or poor environment is difficult to ascertain. However, there are some age-related physiologic changes that all humans experience that affect sleep.

Older adults' sleep architecture—the structure of their sleep cycles—differs from that of younger adults in that they spend less time in the deeper slow-wave sleep stage and have few, briefer episodes of Rapid Eye Movement (REM) sleep. Because older adults spend more time in the earlier, lighter, sleep stages (1 and 2), they can experience a greater numbers of arousals. However, these changes are part of normal changes across the life-span and seem to stabilize after age 60.[7,10,11] In addition, older adults tend to have a flattened circadian rhythm, and experience a "phase advance" (earlier bedtime and early morning awakenings),[8] which may be due to age-related deterioration in the suprachiasmic nucleus, the body's "clock." Some studies have shown that the secretion of melatonin, the hormone secreted by the pineal gland that helps control the daily sleep–wake cycle, is decreased in older adults, which can make it harder to get to sleep. However, these changes are not seen universally. Zeitzer and colleagues[13] found no difference in the endogenous amplitude of plasma melatonin levels and many older people have no sleep complaints. Naylor and Zee[14] suggest that factors other than age, such as comorbidities and levels of light exposure or physical activity, are also important to circadian rhythms changes in older adults.

Chronic Illnesses

As more is understood about the connections between health behaviors, chronic illnesses, and social stresses, researchers have begun to study sleep in conjunction with related physical and psychological complaints. Early sleep assessment instruments asked about pain and nocturia and presence of comorbidities,[15,16] but more recent studies have examined sleep problems as both a symptom of chronic illness and a result of it. Cardiovascular disease, diabetes, chronic obstructive pulmonary disease, depression, and arthritis have been linked strongly with sleep problems in older adults, and more recent studies noted that sleep complaints increase in prevalence with aging in a pattern that tracks the increase in medical conditions and medication use.[17,18] In addition to the discomfort and stress of a chronic condition, many of the medications taken to treat it, including beta-blockers, bronchodilators, calcium channel blockers, corticosteroids, decongestants, stimulating antidepressants, and thyroid hormones, are stimulating and can disrupt sleep.[11,19] The National Sleep Foundation's Sleep in America Survey (2003) found that sleep disturbance and chronic disease—hypertension, arthritis, depression, stroke, diabetes, and chronic obstructive pulmonary disease—go hand in hand.[20] Having a medical disorder significantly increased the likelihood of sleeping fewer than 6 hours a day, having insomnia, or being excessively sleepy during the daytime. And having more than 1 chronic condition increased the likelihood of sleep disorders. Thus, an older adult with painful arthritis is very likely to have trouble sleeping, which can worsen arthritis symptoms.

In one of the most rigorous and frequently cited epidemiologic studies of poor sleep in older adults, 42% of community-dwelling older adults (n = 6899) reported difficulty in initiating and maintaining sleep.[21] In a 3-year follow-up study of these elderly individuals, the authors noted that of the 2000 survivors who had reported chronic difficulties at baseline, about 50% no longer had insomnia symptoms at the 3-year follow-up, and the decrease in sleep complaints was associated with improvement in health. The authors concluded that aging alone does not account for the sleep complaints of the older adult; rather, it is the associated health problems that are associated with poor sleep. Nurses caring for older adults need to consider sleep-related health outcomes when helping patients to manage chronic illnesses.

Psychosocial Stressors

Other important factors to consider when assessing older adults with sleep problems are psychosocial changes that frequently accompany aging. In the general adult population, stressful life events such as a job loss, the arrival of a new baby, or a divorce might cause people to have trouble sleeping until they have adapted to the change or the situation is resolved. However, many of the stressful life events older people experience, such as retirement, bereavement, the onset of chronic illness or disability, or changes of living situation, are perceived as losses or signs of increasing dependency. Moreover, it is common for an older adult to experience many or all of these life changes in different combinations or in fairly rapid succession over a short period of time.[22] Older adults who, for example, move from their own homes to a retirement community, or to assisted living, and in many cases, again to long-term care or a nursing home, are experiencing increasing dependence, a loss of control of personal routines and environment, and the imposition of greater social and physical restrictions. In a chapter in *Case Studies in Insomnia*, on the older adult, Flaxman noted:

> Older insomniacs are likely to be dealing with different life issues than younger insomniacs. Issues such as understanding one's own aging, death and dying, and coping with chronic illness and disability are important for this population (Knight, 1986). For some clients, the stress that these life cycle issues can create must be addressed in treatment, rather than other issues that are more common in a younger population.[23]

It is important to remember to ask about these social issues and possible changes to living situation when talking with older people about sleep problems. In **Fig. 1**, Khan-Hudson and Alessi[24] diagrammed a possible model for the interaction between the physical and psychosocial stressors that can result in sleep problems. In their model, decreasing sleep quality (caused by medical conditions, bereavement, and poor environment) leads to decreased social interaction, decreased cognition, and an increasingly negative self-perception. Improving nighttime sleep, by perhaps eliminating sleep-inhibiting medications, treating medical conditions, relieving pain, and improving sleep hygiene, can have wide-ranging improvements on mental and emotional health, social interaction, and quality of life.[22,23]

DIAGNOSING AND MANAGING SLEEP DISORDERS IN EVERYDAY FUNCTION

Older adults who seek help from nurses about sleep problems often initially complain about insomnia, because it is the most common sleep disorder and one that is familiar to many people. However, it is important for nurses to be aware of other sleep

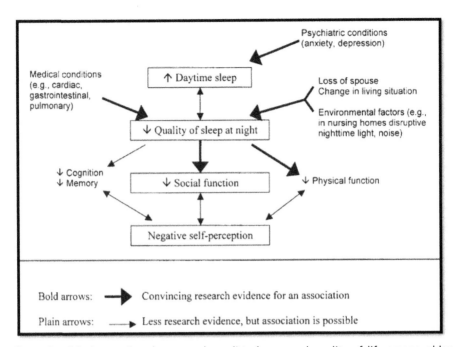

Fig. 1. Possible interactions between sleep disturbance and quality of life among older adults. (*Adapted from*: Khan-Hudson A, Alessi C. Sleep and quality of life in older people. In: Verster J, Pandi-Perumal S, Streiner D, eds. *Sleep and Quality of Life in Clinical Medicine.* Humana Press; 2008:131-138.)

problems that may be causing disrupted sleep, and to differentiate between them. The National Sleep Foundation notes that the discussion of sleep occurs in clinical interviews infrequently, mainly when clients report distressing symptoms related to sleep, such as trouble falling and staying asleep, depression, anxiety, or pain.[20,25] A diagnostic algorithm, like the one in **Fig. 2**, is helpful in guiding differential diagnosis (eg, insomnia, obstructive sleep apnea [OSA], and restless legs syndrome) with different kinds of sleep disruptions, and determining whether the sleep problems are the result of a sleep disorder, or a side effect of another condition or medication.[26]

Insomnia

The most common sleep disorder among older adults is insomnia. Insomnia is characterized by a subjective perception of difficulty initiating or maintaining sleep and can involve difficulty getting to sleep at the beginning of the night, difficulty staying asleep through the night, or premature awakening in the morning with an inability to fall back asleep, associated with significant distress or impairment of daytime functioning.[27–29] Epidemiologic reports of insomnia vary somewhat, depending on the diagnostic criteria used and population assessed, but it is estimated that 10% to 15% of the healthy adult population has chronic insomnia (sleep difficulties lasting more than a month), and an additional 25% to 35% has occasional or transient insomnia.[10,19,21,30] Among older adults (age $\geq$65 years), however, the prevalence rates are much higher, ranging from 25% to 57% for people living in the community to 65% of people living in institutions.[21,29,31]

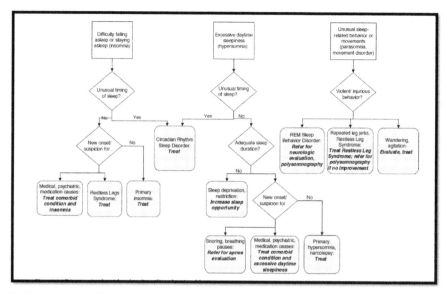

Fig. 2. Diagnostic algorithm for sleep disorders. (Source: "Evidence-based recommendations for the assessment and management of sleep disorders in older persons" by H. G. Bloom, I. Ahmed, C. A. Alessi et al, 2009. *Journal of the American Geriatrics Society, 57, pp 761-789.*)

Chronic insomnia is too often dismissed as an unpleasant consequence of aging, like presbyopia or fragile skin. However, insomnia is both a problem in itself and at the same time can be a symptom of other, potentially serious mental or physical health issues. Multiple research studies have found that insomnia in older adults is linked to an increased incidence of falls,[31,32] depression and anxiety,[33] suicide attempts,[34] cognitive impairment,[35] institutionalization,[36] and overall mortality.[37] Insomnia prevalence increases with age, but the reasons for this increase are complex. Epidemiologic studies of insomnia in older adults in journals and textbooks have used varying methods, diagnostic criteria, and measurements over the last 30 years (**Box 1**) and made varying, sometimes conflicting conclusions about the role of physiologic aging itself.[4,7,19,29] **Fig. 3** shows the increase in the 3 types of insomnia across the lifespan, and how sleep maintenance frequently proves more difficult for older adults.

Treatment for short-term or acute insomnia can include relaxation exercises, improvements in sleep hygiene (**Box 2**) and occasionally a prescription for sleeping medications. However, hypnotic and sedative medications are not recommended for older adults owing to an increased risks of falls and other severe health risks.[38] Treatment for chronic insomnia includes a combination of cognitive behavioral therapy to address any dysfunctional beliefs and attitudes toward sleep combined with education about good sleep hygiene.

Case study: insomnia

Robert is a 78-year-old retired middle school principal, whose wife, Zoe, died 18 months ago. A year before Zoe's death, Robert and Zoe sold their family home in Topeka, Kansas, and moved to an apartment in a retirement community in the suburbs of Dallas, to be near their daughter, Josie, and her family. Robert now lives in the 1-bedroom apartment alone, and Josie visits him several times a week. Robert describes his health as "pretty good for my age." He has arthritis and takes medication

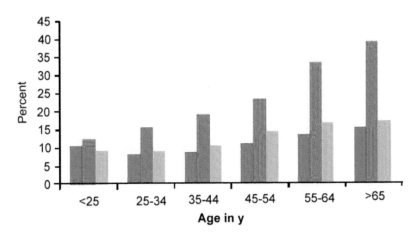

Difficulty initiating   Difficulty maintaining   Early morning awakenings

Fig. 3. Sleep disturbances by type over the lifespan. (*Adapted from* Ohayon, M., & Reynolds, C. (2009). Epidemiological and clinical relevance of insomnia diagnosis algorithms according to the DSM-IV and the International Classification of Sleep Disorders (ICSD). *Sleep Medicine, 10(9), 952–960.*)

for hypertension. When they first moved to the community he still drove during the daytime, but he has not used his car for the last year.

Robert has come to see his health care provider after much urging from his daughter, because he fell asleep at his grandson's baseball game, and Josie was very concerned to learn that her father has been sleeping only 4 to 5 hours a night for many months. Robert's nurse asks him about his sleep routine, caffeine and alcohol intake, and bedroom environment. Robert reports that he is not in pain, that he walks around the retirement community's fitness paths 3 times a week. He says he goes to bed at 11 PM and frequently lies awake until after 1 AM; "I just lie there thinking and I can't turn my brain off," he says. On the nights when he does go to sleep quickly, he often finds himself awake from 3 AM to 5 AM and then sleeps until 10, but is still exhausted the next day. His daughter once told him not to lie in bed if he cannot

---

Box 1
Insomnia diagnostic criteria

One notable change in the last 20 years has been revision of the definition and diagnosis of insomnia in the American Psychiatric Association's *Diagnostic and Statistical Manual*, 5th edition (DSM-5), which was published in 2013. The DSM-5 lists the following criteria for a diagnosis of insomnia:

- The individual experiences dissatisfaction with sleep quantity or quality, with one or more of the following symptoms: difficulty initiating sleep, difficulty maintaining sleep, early morning awakening.
- The sleep disturbance causes significant distress or impairment in social, occupational, educational, academic, behavioral, or other important areas of functioning.
- The sleep difficulty occurs at least 3 nights per week and is present for at least 3 months despite adequate opportunity for sleep.
- The insomnia does not co-occur with another sleep disorder.
- The insomnia is not explained by coexisting mental disorders or medical conditions.[28]

Box 2
Sleep hygiene guidelines from the American Academy of Sleep Medicine[27]

- Keep a consistent sleep schedule. Get up at the same time every day, even on weekends or during vacations.
- Set a bedtime that is, early enough for you to get at least 7 hours of sleep,
- Do not go to bed unless you are sleepy.
- If you do not fall asleep after 20 minutes in bed, get up.
- Establish a relaxing bedtime routine.
- Use your bed only for sleep and sex.
- Make your bedroom quiet and relaxing. Keep the room at a comfortable, cool temperature.
- Limit exposure to bright light in the evenings.
- Turn off electronic devices at least 30 minutes before bedtime.
- Do not eat a large meal before bedtime. If you are hungry at night, eat a light, healthy snack.
- Avoid consuming caffeine in the late afternoon or evening.
- Avoid consuming alcohol before bedtime.
- Decrease your fluid intake before bedtime.

---

sleep, but to get up, so he goes to the living room and does jigsaw puzzles on his iPad until he feels sleepy again. Robert admitted that he is lonely without his wife and misses her presence in bed. He said he keeps the television on in the living room all night because it makes him feel less alone.

His nurse asks him whether he thinks he might be depressed and asks him depression screening questions. Robert admits that he has not enjoyed any social activities at the community for many months and agrees to try 10 mg/d sertraline (Zoloft) and to call a therapist to talk about grief counseling. His nurse also talks to him about sleep hygiene and ways to get himself to sleep better. They agree a 2-week sleep plan, which involves getting up at the same time every day, drinking no caffeine after 11 AM, using the sleep setting on his clock radio instead of the TV, to decrease noise in the apartment, and completing a sleep diary for 14 nights. On the next visit, Robert reports that he has been sleeping 6 to 8 hours per night and that he feels much more energetic. He found a therapist who is teaching him cognitive behavioral therapy techniques to quiet his mind and find outlets for his memories of Zoe, and is encouraged with his progress.

Obstructive Sleep Apnea

OSA is the most common sleep-related breathing disorder in older adults, and frequently leads to significant impairments in sleep quality and daytime functioning.[39] OSA is characterized by frequent obstruction of the upper airway during sleep, which leads to oxyhemoglobin desaturation, arousals or fragmented sleep. OSA severity is measured with the apnea-hypopnea index (AHI), which refers to the number of apneas that occur during an hour of sleep. An apnea is defined as a cessation ($\geq$90% decrease in breathing) for at least 10 seconds during sleep.[39] These arousals and episodes of hypoxia lead to daytime symptoms such as fatigue, impaired cognition, and drowsiness.

OSA is a very common cause of disrupted sleep. Approximately 24% of people over the age of 65 had an AHI of 5 or higher, and 62% had an AHI of 10 events per hour or more.[39] Patients with untreated OSA typically present with reports of snoring and restless sleep. A detailed physical assessment that includes anthropometric measures including height, weight, body mass index, waist–hip ratio, and neck circumference can help to identify risk factors for OSA[40] and reports from bed partners about snoring and any witnessed apneas are helpful. However, a diagnosis requires a polysomnographic study. Polysomnography used to require an overnight stay in a sleep laboratory, but new in-home test kits are becoming more affordable and have been shown to give reliable results.

Treatment for OSA includes continuous positive airway pressure (CPAP) therapy, oral appliances, weight loss, and surgical treatments, depending on the patient's physiology.[39] CPAP involves the delivery of positive air pressure through a nasal or full-face mask, worn in bed every night. CPAP decreases desaturations and apneic episodes, but patients must wear it consistently. Adherence to treatment is problematic for many patients, who complain about noise and discomfort of the device, but encouragement and support from family and health care providers in the first weeks can be influential as the patient begins to see improvements in sleep quality and daytime energy levels.[40] Oral appliances can be used for patients with mild to moderate OSA, or those who prefer them to CPAP, do not respond to CPAP, are not candidates for CPAP, or fail treatment attempts with CPAP or behavioral measures (such as weight loss or sleep position change).[40]

Case study: obstructive sleep apnea

Marco Perez, age 70, is a history professor at a small college. He has type 2 diabetes, which he controls fairly well with diet. He is often sleepy during the day and his partner, Simon, has complained about Marco's snoring for many years, and occasionally slept in another room when it got intolerable. But after seeing a documentary about sleep apnea online, Simon realized that what he had been observing alongside Marco's snoring were apneic episodes. He became very concerned about the possible long-term effects of OSA, including heart attack and stroke, and urged Marco to see a sleep specialist. Marco agreed and underwent a polysomnography sleep study which indicated a respiratory disturbance index of 34 per hour with 51 desaturations of less than 90%, while supine. The longest event that occurred was a 32-second period of obstructive apnea with a decrease in oxygen saturation to 86%. The sleep clinic recommended CPAP, and although Marco was worried about the noise and embarrassed to wear the mask, he agreed to try it for 3 weeks. Simon assured him that the CPAP was manageable and encouraged him to seek help from the equipment provider and clinic staff until he was comfortable with the fit. At the end of the 3-week trial Marco and Simon reported that they were able to sleep together comfortably, and that Marco had more energy during the day.

Review of Novel Interventions for Sleep Promotion

Many older adults with sleep problems seek help from health care providers only after trying to manage the problem themselves for some time. Many traditional or folkloric remedies are still used informally despite there being little empirical evidence for their efficacy.[41] Herbal teas, aromatherapy, hot baths, massages, and other procedures may work by calming and relaxing the mind and preparing the person to sleep and are reasonable components of a bedtime routine if combined with other types of sleep hygiene. Improving sleep hygiene, the personal habits and environmental factors that affect sleep quality, is often the first step in improving sleep.[30,32,40]

A number of intervention studies have tested the effects of alternative or complementary therapies on older adults' sleep. Yoga,[42] acupressure,[43] Tai Chi,[44] and mindfulness meditation[45] have all been shown to improve older adults' scores on the Pittsburgh Sleep Quality Index. In a rigorous systematic review of insomnia and complementary medicine and therapies, Sarris and Byrne[41] found good empirical support for traditional Indo-Asian therapies—Tai Chi, acupuncture, acupressure, and yoga—but less for common Western complementary and alternative therapies, such as homeopathy, valerian, or massage. Two other types of alternative therapies—exercise programs and bright light exposure—have also been tested, but with mixed results.[46] Exercise programs have focused on good sleepers or younger adults, leaving little room for measuring improvements in older people. Research into bright light therapy has been concentrated on people living with dementia in institutions where they have decrease exposure to daylight. There have been encouraging results in using bright light exposure to synchronize disturbed sleep and reduce frequency of behavior disorders,[47,48] but more research is needed.

Future Directions for Sleep Research

Nursing practice would benefit from a greater awareness of the importance of sleep to all sectors of the population. Many nursing textbooks address sleep only in the context of certain diseases (Alzheimer's disease, cancer). However, the issue is especially important when nursing older adults. Too often, ageist stereotypes about sleep habits blind health care providers to real issues in physical and mental health and lead to unnecessary suffering. When assessing sleep in older adults, nurses must not simply ask, "How are you sleeping?" but probe further to determine sleep duration, number of awakenings, napping habits, and how patients feel about their sleep. Older adults, too, may have accepted the stereotype that poor sleep comes with age and not tell their health care provider because it is not as big a problem as their cardiovascular disease, diabetes, or arthritis. Health care providers need to be aware that sleep affects the whole person and can have as much impact on the trajectory and management of their chronic disease as the proper medications or treatment.

CLINICS CARE POINTS

- Contrary to popular beliefs about aging, research has shown that healthy older adults and younger adults require comparable amounts of sleep, but that multiple health, social, and environmental risk factors make achieving that need much more difficult as people age.

- Improving nighttime sleep, by perhaps eliminating sleep-inhibiting medications, treating medical conditions, relieving pain, and improving sleep hygiene, can have wide-ranging improvements on mental and emotional health, social interaction, and quality of life.[22,23]

- Treatment for short-term or acute insomnia can include relaxation exercises, improvements in sleep hygiene, and occasionally a prescription for sleeping medications. However, hypnotic and sedative medications are not generally recommended for older adults owing to the increased risk for falls and other severe health risks.

- Improving sleep hygiene, the personal habits and environmental factors that affect sleep quality, is often the first step in improving sleep.

- When assessing sleep in older adults, nurses must not simply ask, "How are you sleeping?" but probe further to determine sleep duration, number of awakenings, napping habits, and how patients feel about their sleep.

REFERENCES

1. Pandi-Perumal S, Monti J, Monjan A, editors. Principles and practice of geriatric sleep medicine. Cambridge (UK): Cambridge University Press; 2010.

2. An C, Yu L, Wang L, et al. Association between sleep characteristics and mild cognitive impairment in elderly people. Neurophysiology 2014;46(1):88–94.
3. Tsapanou A, Gu Y, O'Shea D, et al. Daytime somnolence as an early sign of cognitive decline in a community-based study of older people: daytime somnolence and cognitive decline. Int J Geriatr Psychiatry 2016;31(3):247–55.
4. Ancoli-Israel S. Sleep and aging: prevalence of disturbed sleep and treatment considerations in older adults. J Clin Psychiatry 2004;66(Suppl 9):24–30.
5. Jaussent I, Bouyer J, Ancelin M-L, et al. Insomnia and daytime sleepiness are risk factors for depressive symptoms in the elderly. Sleep 2011;34(8):1103–10.
6. Institute of Medicine. In: Colten H, editor. Sleep disorders and sleep deprivation: an unmet public health problem. 1st edition. Washington, DC: National Academies Press; 2006.
7. Morin C, Espie C. Insomnia: a clinical guide to assessment and treatment. New York: Springer Publishing Company; 2004.
8. Redeker N. Developmental aspects of normal sleep. In: Redeker N, McEnany G, editors. Sleep disorders and sleep promotion in nursing practice. New York: Springer Publishing Company; 2011. p. 19–32.
9. Hirshkowitz M, Whiton K, Albert SM, et al. National Sleep Foundation's sleep time duration recommendations: methodology and results summary. Sleep Health J Natl Sleep Found 2015;1(1):40–3.
10. Petrov M, Vander Wal G, Lichstein K. Late-life insomnia. In: Pachana N, Pachana N, Laidlaw K, et al, editors. The oxford handbook of clinical geropsychology. Oxford Library of Psychology. New York: Oxford University Press; 2014. p. 527–48.
11. Ancoli-Israel S, Cooke J. Prevalence and comorbidity of insomnia and effect on functioning in elderly populations. J Am Geriatr Soc 2005;53(S7):S264–71.
12. Ruiter M, Vander Wal G, Lichstein K. Insomnia in the elderly. In: Pandi-Perumal S, Monti J, Monjan A, editors. Geriatric sleep medicine. New York: Cambridge University Press; 2010. p. 271–9.
13. Zeitzer J, Daniels J, Duffy J. Do plasma melatonin concentrations decline with age? Am J Med 1999;107(5):432–6.
14. Naylor E, Zee P. Circadian rhythm sleep disorders in aging. In: Avidan A, Alessi C, editors. Geriatric sleep medicine. New York: Informa Healthcare; 2008. p. 179–95.
15. Buysse DJ, Reynolds CF, Monk TH, et al. The Pittsburgh sleep quality index: a new instrument for psychiatric practice and research. Psychiatry Res 1989; 28(2):193–213.
16. Rombaut N, Maillard F, Kelly F, et al. The quality of life of insomniacs questionnaire (QOLI). Med Sci Res 1990;18:845–7.
17. Foley D, Ancoli-Israel S, Britz P, et al. Sleep disturbances and chronic disease in older adults. J Psychosom Res 2004;56(5):497–502.
18. Barczi S. Sleep and medical comorbidities. In: Avidan A, Alessi C, editors. Geriatric sleep medicine. New York: Informa Healthcare; 2008. p. 19–36.
19. Ohayon M. Epidemiology of insomnia: what we know and what we still need to learn. Sleep Med Rev 2002;6(2):97–111.
20. National Sleep Foundation. 2003 sleep in America poll. 2003. Available at: https://sleepfoundation.org/sites/default/files/2003SleepPollExecSumm.pdf. Accessed October 12, 2020.
21. Foley D, Monjan A, Brown S, et al. Sleep complaints among elderly persons: an epidemiologic study of three communities. Sleep 1995;18(6):425–32.

22. Berkley A, Carter P, Yoder L, et al. The effects of insomnia on older adults' quality of life and daily functioning: a mixed-methods study. Geriatr Nurs 2020;41(6): 832–8.

23. Flaxman J. Insomnia in the older adult. In: Hauri P, editor. Case studies in insomnia. New York: Plenum Publishing Co; 1991. p. 237–47.

24. Khan-Hudson A, Alessi C. Sleep and quality of life in older people. In: Verster J, Pandi-Perumal S, Streiner D, editors. Sleep and quality of life in clinical medicine. Totowa (NJ): Humana Press; 2008. p. 131–8.

25. Cole C. Sleep and primary care of adults and older adults. In: Redeker N, McEnany G, editors. Sleep disorders and sleep promotion in nursing practice. New York: Springer Publishing Company; 2011. p. 291–308.

26. Bloom HG, Ahmed I, Alessi CA, et al. Evidence-based recommendations for the assessment and management of sleep disorders in older persons. J Am Geriatr Soc 2009;57(5):761–89.

27. American Academy of Sleep Medicine. International classification of sleep disorders. 3rd edition. Darien (IL): American Academy of Sleep Medicine; 2014.

28. American Psychiatric Association. Diagnostic and statistical manual of mental disorders. 5th edition. Washington, DC: American Psychiatric Publishing; 2013.

29. Voyer P, Verreault R, Mengue PN, et al. Prevalence of insomnia and its associated factors in elderly long-term care residents. Arch Gerontol Geriatr 2006; 42(1):1–20.

30. Benca R. Diagnosis and treatment of chronic insomnia: a review. Psychiatr Serv 2005;56(3):332–43.

31. Martin J, Ancoli-Israel S. Sleep disturbances in long-term care. Clin Geriatr Med 2008;24(1):39, vi.

32. Krishnan P, Hawranik P. Diagnosis and management of geriatric insomnia: a guide for nurse practitioners. J Am Acad Nurse Pract 2008;20(12):590–9.

33. Potvin O, Lorrain D, Belleville G, et al. Subjective sleep characteristics associated with anxiety and depression in older adults: a population-based study. Int J Geriatr Psychiatry 2014;29(12):1262–70.

34. Bernert RA, Turvey CL, Conwell Y, et al. Association of poor subjective sleep quality with risk for death by suicide during a 10-year period: a longitudinal, population-based study of late life. JAMA Psychiatry 2014;71(10):1129–37.

35. Almondes KM de, Costa MV, Malloy-Diniz LF, et al. Insomnia and risk of dementia in older adults: systematic review and meta-analysis. J Psychiatr Res 2016;77: 109–15.

36. Pollak C, Perlick D. Sleep problems and institutionalization of the elderly. Top Geriatr 1991;4(4):204–10.

37. Dew M, Hoch C, Buysse D, et al. Healthy older adults' sleep predicts all-cause mortality at 4-19 years follow-up. Psychosom Med 2003;65:63–73.

38. Sateia M, Buysse D, Krystal A, et al. Clinical practice guideline for the pharmacologic treatment of chronic insomnia in adults: an American Academy of Sleep Medicine clinical practice guideline. J Clin Sleep Med 2017;13(2):307–49.

39. Gooneratne N. Sleep-related breathing disorders in aging. In: Avidan A, Alessi C, editors. Geriatric sleep medicine. New York: Informa Healthcare; 2008. p. 141–56.

40. Case study: obstructive sleep apnea. - Free Online Library. Available at: https://www.thefreelibrary.com/Case+study%3a+obstructive+sleep+apnea.-a0176372182. Accessed October 19, 2020.

41. Sarris J, Byrne GJ. A systematic review of insomnia and complementary medicine. Sleep Med Rev 2011;15(2):99–106.

42. Halpern J, Cohen M, Kennedy G, et al. Yoga for improving sleep quality and quality of life for older adults. Altern Ther Health Med 2014;20(3):37–46.

43. Lai F, Chen I, Chen P, et al. Acupressure, sleep, and quality of life in institutionalized older adults: a randomized controlled trial. J Am Geriatr Soc 2017. https://doi.org/10.1111/jgs.14729.

44. Chan AW, Yu DS, Choi KC, et al. Tai chi qigong as a means to improve night-time sleep quality among older adults with cognitive impairment: a pilot randomized controlled trial. Clin Interv Aging 2016;11:1277–86.

45. Black DS, O'Reilly GA, Olmstead R, et al. Mindfulness meditation and improvement in sleep quality and daytime impairment among older adults with sleep disturbances: a randomized clinical trial. JAMA Intern Med 2015;175(4):494–501.

46. Montgomery P, Dennis J. A systematic review of non-pharmacological therapies for sleep problems in later life. Sleep Med Rev 2004;8(1):47–62.

47. Friedman L, Spira AP, Hernandez B, et al. Brief morning light treatment for sleep/wake disturbances in older memory-impaired individuals and their caregivers. Sleep Med 2012;13(5):546–9.

48. Benloucif S, Green K, L'Hermite-Balériaux M, et al. Responsiveness of the aging circadian clock to light. Neurobiol Aging 2006;27(12):1870–9.

Sleep Assessment for Sleep Problems in Children

Laurie A. Martinez, PhD, MBA, MSN, RN[a],*,
Shannon M. Constantinides, PhD, MSN, FNP, NP-C, RN[b]

KEYWORDS

- Sleep • Sleep assessment • Sleep problems • Children

KEY POINTS

- Sleep problems are common in children and may affect biopsychosocial health, emotional and behavioral regulation, immune function, mental health, cognition, development, and productivity.
- Sleep and thorough sleep assessments are often overlooked in routine health assessments and sleep problems often go unrecognized.
- Nurses are well positioned to assess, identify, and address sleep problems and positively impact childhood health, development, and overall well-being.

INTRODUCTION

Sleep is an active process with varying functions that differ with age and development, and are inclusive of, but not limited to, brain development,[1] synaptic plasticity,[2,3] learning and attention,[4] emotional regulation,[5] and behavior.[6] Neurologic structures responsible for sleep processes develop during the first few years of life.[7] Literature has demonstrated that sleep disruption may alter sleep processes and negatively impact cognition, emotion, and behavior.[2–6,8] Of concern are the results from studies that have reported up to 50% of children experience sleep problems and 4% of children are estimated to live with a diagnosable sleep disorder.[9,10] Although sleep disruptions are common during childhood, identification of childhood sleep problems is easily missed because they may present differently when compared with adults.[11] For example, although adults with sleep problems may present with overt sleepiness, children with sleep problems may present with hyperactivity, inattentiveness, learning struggles, mood swings, frustration, and/or irritation.[12,13] Unless sleep problems in children are severe, there is a low rate of parents reporting these issues to health care providers, because most parents are unaware of the relationship between sleep deprivation and daytime behaviors.[14] Processes to screen for sleep problems is

[a] Florida Atlantic University, Christine E. Lynn College of Nursing, 777 Glades Road, Boca Raton, FL 33431, USA; [b] Colorado Center of Orthopedic Excellence, 2446 Research Parkway, Suite 200, Colorado Springs, CO 80920, USA
* Corresponding author.
E-mail address: Lauriemartin2017@health.fau.edu

Nurs Clin N Am 56 (2021) 299–309
https://doi.org/10.1016/j.cnur.2021.02.008
0029-6465/21/© 2021 Elsevier Inc. All rights reserved.

critical because early identification may nurture and improve biopsychosocial development.[1–8] Likewise, screening has the potential to identify children who may need or benefit from interdisciplinary diagnostic testing resulting in prevention of developmental delays and complications associated with poor sleep, sleep problems, and diagnosable sleep disorders.[15]

This article provides education for clinicians on childhood sleep problems, including an overview of the cause and natural course of sleep problems if left untreated, strategies for accurate sleep-related history taking, and when to refer patients for further testing or to a higher or more specialized level of care. Although a brief overview of diagnosable sleep disorders and diagnostic tests for child sleep disorders is presented (**Table 1**), note that the breadth of childhood sleep disorders is broad and includes a multidisciplinary approach from screening through treatment. An in-depth discussion of diagnosable sleep disorders is beyond the scope of this paper.

SLEEP ASSESSMENT

Sleep, as a function of health, and thorough sleep assessments can often be overlooked in routine health assessments.[19] This is of concern because sleep impacts childhood biopsychosocial health and is associated with emotional and behavioral regulation, immune function, mental health, cognition, development, and productivity.[1–8,16,20,21] Identifying and addressing sleep problems has potential to optimize childhood health. Nurses are positioned well to recognize potential sleep problems by incorporating sleep questions within routine child health assessments. A sleep assessment can identify child sleep problems and provide insight if further sleep evaluation is warranted for sleep disorders (see **Table 1**). The following sections provide guidance on performing a childhood sleep history within the context of a general health history.

Sleep History

The sleep history captures information about a child's sleep routines and schedules, sleep initiation and maintenance, sleep movements and behaviors, respiratory problems, and daytime sleepiness and behaviors.[22–24]

Sleep routines and sleep schedules

Evening routines and sleep-wake schedules are essential for optimal sleep. To identify potential sleep problems, nurses should inquire about sleep routines and schedules, including events that happen before bedtime, at bedtime, on awaking, and events on awaking. Knowledge of bedtimes and hours of sleep, caregiver perspectives on appropriate bedtimes and hours of sleep, consistency with sleep routines and schedules, and types of activities the child is engaged with before bed (ie, homework, television, video games, reading) can provide insight into potential sleep problems (**Table 2** for recommended required sleep).[23] Nurses should inquire about consistency of sleep schedules, presence of parents or siblings during sleep initiation, potential environmental sleep disruptors (ie, sharing a room; living in a loud apartment building; outside noise, such as traffic; screens in room), and responses of parent or caregiver when child stalls before bed.[23] Additionally, specific types and times of activities (ie, sports, homework, dinner) along with screen usage (ie, television, electronic devices) should be assessed and noted because recent research has indicated that screen usage is associated with delayed sleep initiation[28] and decreased sleep duration.[29]

Note that if a parent presents with concerns about a child's sleep, they frequently report what have been the most recent or most severe sleep experiences. As such, it is pertinent nurses inquire about frequency, duration, and variability of sleep and

Table 1
Childhood sleep disorders with associated conditions and diagnostic testing

Sleep Disorder Category	Brief Description of Sleep Disorder Category	Potential Conditions and Disorders Associated with Sleep Problems	Diagnostic and Monitoring Tools
Insomnias	Sleep initiation and sleep maintenance difficulties	Colic; gastroesophageal reflux; food allergies; pain, enuresis; psychosocial factors; parental smoking; night wakings; ADHD; autism; obesity	Sleep diary, nocturnal polysomnography, daytime multiple sleep latency test, maintenance of wakefulness test, dim light melatonin onset, actigraphy, parent and self-reported sleep surveys and questionnaires
Hypersomnias	Excessive daytime sleepiness	Narcolepsy, idiopathic hypersomnia, Kleine-Levin syndrome and recurrent hypersomnia, post-traumatic and postneurosurgical hypersomnia, pharmacologic-related hypersomnia	
Sleep and breathing disorders	Airway dysfunction during sleep that causes increased respiratory efforts	Apnea, apparent life-threatening events, primary snoring, obstructive sleep apnea	
Parasomnias	Undesirable events that occur during sleep	Sleep-related dissociative disorders, enuresis, sleep-related groaning, sleep-related eating disorder, parasomnia caused by medical condition	
Movement disorders	Simple sleep-related nocturnal movements	Rhythmic movement disorder, sleep-related bruxism, restless leg syndrome, periodic limb movement	

(continued on next page)

Table 1 (continued)			
Sleep Disorder Category	Brief Description of Sleep Disorder Category	Potential Conditions and Disorders Associated with Sleep Problems	Diagnostic and Monitoring Tools
Sleep in medical disorders and special populations	At risk for increased frequency of sleep disturbance when compared with healthy peers	Epilepsy, cancer, bipolar disorder, depression, anxiety, obsessive-compulsive disorder, PTSD, allergic rhinitis, asthma, chronic pain conditions, craniofacial abnormalities, cystic fibrosis, gastroesophageal reflux, sickle cell disease, food allergies, rheumatologic conditions	

Abbreviations: ADHD, attention-deficit/hyperactivity disorder; PTSD, post-traumatic stress disorder.
Data gathered and compiled for table format from Refs.[16–18]

Table 2 Sleep requirements for children and adolescents with common sleep problems		
Age	Hours of Recommended Sleep	Sleep Problems
1–2 y	11–14 (including naps)	Bedtime resistance, night awakenings, rhythmic movements
3–5 y	10–13 h (including naps)	Bedtime resistance, night awakenings, apnea, rhythmic movements, sleepwalking, confusional arousal, sleep terrors, nightmares
6–12 y	9–12 h	Inadequate sleep, unhealthy sleep hygiene, behavioral insomnia, sleepwalking, confusional arousal, sleep terrors, nightmares, apnea, restless leg syndrome
13–18 y	8–10 h	Inadequate sleep, unhealthy sleep hygiene, daytime sleepiness, delayed sleep phase, apnea, behavioral insomnia, restless leg syndrome

Data gathered and compiled for table format from Refs.[25–27] sleep concerns from day to day, looking longitudinally for sleep patterns.[24] Additionally, if a child has a history of sleep problems, nurses should note interventions, treatments (pharmacologic and nonpharmacologic), and strategies that were tried, and include outcomes of the interventions as perceived by the parent and child.

Several valid sleep checklists and questionnaires exist to assist nurses when a more detailed sleep history is warranted (ie, Pediatric Daytime Sleepiness Scale, Epworth Sleepiness Scale for Children, Children's Sleep Hygiene Scale). Of specific relevance to nurses performing sleep history is the BEARS screening questionnaire.[30] The BEARS questionnaire assesses five sleep domains: (1) bedtime, (2) excessive daytime sleepiness, (3) awakenings at night, (4) regularity/duration, and (5) snoring. Although it has no diagnostic power it can assist nurses in identifying children in need of further sleep evaluation.[30] Note that checklists and questionnaires are not meant to replace the sleep history but rather enhance data gathered from the sleep history.

Sleep initiation and maintenance
Assessment related to sleep-onset latency (SOL) and night waking are necessary for evaluation of potential sleep problems versus sleep disorders, and for identifying potential differential diagnosis. SOL is the amount of time it takes a child to fall asleep. SOL of 30 minutes or more is considered problematic.[23] Combining SOL and night waking with the child's sleep history (behavior, evening activities, bedtime routines, bedtime schedules) can identify concerning sleep patterns related to psychological, circadian, behavioral, and/or medical issues that may warrant further investigation.[24] Such issues may include anxiety, insomnia, or circadian rhythm sleep-wake disorder. Assessment should include where the child falls asleep (ie, parents bed, child's bed, sofa) and if anyone or anything is with the child when falling asleep (ie, television, music, parent, sibling).[23] For example, when a child can fall asleep with ease in front of the television but struggles to initiate sleep when in their bed may suggest a behavioral sleep etiology because medical origins create prolonged sleep initiation no matter where the child is, who they are with, or what they are surrounded by. Similarly, nurses should assess frequency and duration of child nighttime awakenings and inquire about parental responses to determine if awakenings are influenced by psychological, circadian, behavioral, or medical causes.

Sleep movements and sleep behaviors
An assessment of childhood sleep movements and sleep behaviors is essential in identifying nocturnal movements and behaviors that place the child at risk for injury. Common nocturnal movements include hypnic jerks and hypnagogic foot tremors that occur during childhood and adolescent sleep onset.[31] Sleep-related rhythmic movement disorders usually occur in toddlers, are overall benign (ie, body rocking), and resolve by 5 years old.[32] Although sleep disorder diagnosis is outside the scope of this article, parasomnias warrant brief discussion because these nocturnal behaviors, common in young children, may present risk injuries (ie, sleep walking, confusional arousal).[33] Nurses should inquire about nocturnal episodes of mental confusion, sleepwalking, and inconsolable agitation or screaming. If such behaviors exist, further inquiry should include time and duration of episode (parasomnias usually occur in first third of the night), child recollection of the event, familial patterns, and concerning risks encountered by child associated with such events.[33] Triggers for such events are sleep deprivation; as such, reflection on sleep routines and schedules is of paramount importance. Because parents are usually not with children when sleeping, nurses should empower children to share any sleep concerns they have related to sleep initiation and sleep maintenance by asking about consistent annoying

or concerning behaviors or movements at night or on awakening. Subjective child reports in combination with parental reports are usually adequate to identify potential sleep disorders and to warrant referral for additional diagnostic testing if indicated.

Respiratory problems

Obstructive sleep apnea (OSA) is a common school-aged sleep disorder for children living with obesity, adenotonsillar hypertrophy, and possibly asthma.[34] OSA is characterized by increased nocturnal respiratory efforts and/or snoring and is placed within four categories: (1) primary snoring, (2) upper airway resistance, (3) partial/complete obstruction of upper airway, and (4) obstructive hypoventilation.[34] OSA has long been associated with daytime sleepiness, irritability, decreased school performance, mood swings, and morning headaches.[35] Nurses can assess for OSA by inquiring about daytime sleepiness, sleep restlessness, nocturnal mouth breathing, chronic snoring, chronic respiratory efforts, and parental observed apnea. Children who present with OSA symptoms should be referred to a specialist (ie, otolaryngologist) for further evaluation.

Daytime sleepiness and daytime behavior

The purpose of assessing daytime sleepiness with associated behaviors is to uncover uneasily recognized sleep problems and to identify potential causes of such sleep problems. Often, parents are unaware of age-required sleep and may not associate daytime behaviors with sleep deprivation. As such, all children should be assessed for adequate sleep by merging information gathered from sleep routines, schedules, initiation, maintenance, and inquiries about daytime sleepiness and behaviors. **Table 1** shows sleep requirements recommended by the American Academy of Pediatrics.[25] Nurses should consider and take note of the child's general health, daily physical activities, sleep duration, and quality of sleep when assessing for adequate sleep, along with queries related to daytime sleepiness and associated daytime behaviors. According to the literature, up to half of youth report daytime sleepiness[25] with most not fulfilling the recommended American Academy of Pediatrics nightly hours and approximately 80% experiencing chronic sleep deprivation.[36] It is important to remember that not all children present with sleepiness when struggling with sleep problems; rather, children may present with daytime behavioral issues, such as problems in school or low grades,[37] inattentiveness and emotional dysregulation,[38] and learning problems coupled with anxiety,[39] and increased adolescent risk behaviors (ie, sexual behaviors, safety behaviors).[40] Alternately, many sleep disorders may present with daytime sleepiness (ie, narcolepsy, OSA); as such, concerning sleep patterns may warrant referral to a sleep specialist.

Medical History: Chronic Illness, Developmental and Psychiatric History

Chronic illness

Research has indicated that children with acute or chronic medical conditions experience more sleep problems than children without acute or chronic medical conditions.[16] Literature has also indicated that children with chronic medical conditions experience sleep problems, which may include comorbid sleep disorders, or sleep problems secondary to pharmacologic or interventional treatments and/or hospitalizations.[16] Left untreated, sleep problems may hinder optimal well-being and quality of life by worsening medical conditions; or conversely, exacerbate medical symptoms that may contribute to poor sleep.[16] Therefore, nurses should identify children with chronic medical conditions, particularly those that have the potential to disrupt sleep (ie, juvenile rheumatoid arthritis, epilepsy, cancer, cystic fibrosis, gastroesophageal reflux disease) and inquire about interventions used to treat the medical condition, and if treatments negatively influence sleep.[23]

Developmental and psychiatric history

Children with neurodevelopmental disorders (ie, autism spectrum disorder, attention-deficit/hyperactivity disorder) often experience sleep problems and as such, these conditions are considered a significant comorbidity when considering risk for sleep problems or sleep disorders.[41] Similarly, psychiatric disorders (ie, anxiety, depression) have a high prevalence of sleep problems that include prolonged SOL, short sleep duration, and frequent nighttime awakenings.[42] As such, assessing sleep problems in children with neurodevelopmental and psychiatric disorders is essential because untreated chronic sleep problems within these populations may hinder neurobehavioral functions.[42]

Physical Examination

Nurses are well positioned to perform a thorough physical examination to assess potential physicality indicative of sleep problems. Although the extent of the physical examination depends on the sleep history and presented sleep complaints, nurses should be particularly cognizant of areas related to the airway.[43] **Table 3** provides a general overview of common areas for sleep evaluation.

Table 3
General overview for physical examination within a sleep assessment

General observations	Level of alertness
	Tired eyes
	Frequent position changes
	Hyperactivity
	Frequent yawning
	Sluggishness
	Irritability
Evaluation of growth	Excessive weight gain and/or obesity
Dysmorphic features	Facial asymmetry
	Midface hypoplasia
Craniofacial anomalies	Macrocephaly/microcephaly
	Macrognathia/micrognathia
	Mandibular hypoplasia
Oropharynx and airway	Tonsillar, adenoidal, and/or uvular enlargement
	Oropharyngeal crowding
	Small upper airway
	Mouth breathing
	Noisy breathing
	High-arched palate
	Presence of cleft palate
	Overbite
	Absent gag reflex
	Dysphagia
Neurology	Hypotonia/hypertonia
	Spasticity
	Delayed biopsychosocial development
	Delayed cognitive function
Thorax	Scoliosis
	Pectus excavatum
	Barrel-shaped

Data gathered and compiled to table format from Refs.[17,18]

Box 1
Behavioral strategies to address sleep problems

Sleep Education

- Impact of sleep on brain growth, development, academic performance, emotional and behavioral regulation, learning, and attention
- Sleep requirements per American Academy of Pediatrics guidelines

Sleep Hygiene

- Establish a consistent bedtime and wake time with no more than one difference for weekdays and weekends
- Establish a calm and relaxing bedtime routine 30 minutes immediately before bedtime (ie, reading, meditate, soothing music)
- Avoid using electronic media devices for at least 1 hour before bedtime (ie, televisions, laptop computers, smartphones)
- Create an environment conducive for sleep (quiet, no screens, dark room or low night-light)
- Keep child's bedroom at a comfortable temperature for sleep, approximately 65°F
- Do not use child's bedroom for punishment
- Make sure child is not hungry when going to bed, offer light healthy snacks (ie, yogurt, nuts, fruits; heavy meals within an hour or 2 of bedtime may interfere with sleep)
- Exercise frequently but avoid before bed
- Enjoy the outdoors regularly because sunshine assists internal clock
- Avoid naps for children who are having trouble falling asleep at bedtime
- No caffeine within 6 hours of bed (ie, sodas, iced tea, tea, coffee, chocolate)

Sleep Log

- Track sleep for 2 weeks (1 day = 24 hours)
- Document time child is in bed
- Document time child is sleeping
- Document night awakenings
- Document time awake in the morning
- Assess sleep log and use it to set goals

Sleep Diary

- Use diary to track progress and monitor adherence to plan to reach goal
- Write down the time child got into bed
- Write down the time child tried to go to sleep
- Write down how long it took the child to fall asleep
- Write down the amount of night awakenings
- Write down the time child woke in the morning
- Write down the time child got out of bed in the morning
- Rate quality of sleep: Likert scale
- Write down additional notes about quality of sleep and what may have affected sleep

Box crafted from data derived from Refs.[44,45]

NURSING IMPLICATIONS IN THE CLINICAL SETTING

Nurses who care for and work with children in the clinical setting are well positioned to assess childhood sleep patterns, identify concerning sleep problems, and educate families on the significance of adequate sleep. Assessing for and identifying child sleep problems provides an opportunity for nurses to not only identify rarely recognized sleep problems but also make referrals to specialists for diagnostic testing as warranted. Additionally, performing thorough sleep assessments provides opportunity for the nurse to provide invaluable education to the parent and child on the adverse consequences of sleep deprivation (ie, effects on cognition, emotion, behavior, and school performance). Nurses should take this opportunity to teach the significance of healthy sleep patterns and optimal sleep hygiene. Sleep hygiene encompasses environmental factors and personal habits that affect overall sleep. Strong sleep hygiene promotes daytime, bedtime, and within-sleep practices that facilitate uninterrupted sleep and optimizes sleep-wake transitions.[17] If unhealthy sleep hygiene is identified during the assessment, the nurse should suggest tailored and appropriate behavioral strategies to facilitate sleep. **Box 1** provides an overview of brief behavioral strategies for sleep problems.

SUMMARY

The breadth of childhood sleep issues is broad and is associated with biologic, psychiatric, behavioral, social, and environmental processes. Unrecognized childhood sleep problems may threaten daytime behaviors and negatively impact school and psychosocial functioning. Left unattended, overall biopsychosocial development may be impaired. Thus, identifying and addressing sleep problems has potential to optimize childhood health, development, and overall well-being. Nurses need to be cognizant of detrimental impacts of child sleep deprivation and advocate for appropriate sleep assessments while offering sleep education to parents and children.

CLINICS CARE POINTS

- Most parents do not report child sleep problems as they are unaware of the relationship between sleep deprivation and daytime behaviors.
- Nurses should incorporate sleep questions within routine child health assessments to identify child sleep problems and provide education to the parent and child on the significance of sleep hygiene.
- If unhealthy sleep hygiene is identified by the nurse during the assessment, the nurse should suggest tailored and appropriate behavioral strategies to facilitate sleep.
- The nurse should provide insight if further sleep evaluation is warranted from interdisciplinary diagnostic testing to prevent developmental delays and complications associated with poor sleep, sleep problems, and diagnosable sleep disorders.

DISCLAIMER

The authors have nothing to disclose.

REFERENCES

1. Frank MG. Sleep and developmental plasticity not just for kids. Prog Brain Res 2011;193:221–32.

2. Yoo SS, Gujar N, Hu P, et al. The human emotional brain without sleep: a prefron-tal amygdala disconnect. Curr Biol 2007;17:877–8.

3. eBarnes D, Wilson DA. Sleep and olfactory cortical plasticity. Front Behav Neuro-sci 2014;8:134.

4. Beebe DW, Field J, Miller MM, et al. Impact of multi-night experimentally induced short sleep on adolescent performance in a simulated classroom. Sleep 2017; 40(2):zsw035.

5. Bolinger E, Born J, Zinke K. Sleep divergently affects cognitive and automatic emotional response in children. Neuropsychologia 2018;117:84–91.

6. Telzer EH, Funligni AJ, Lieberman MD, et al. The effects of poor-quality sleep on brain function and risk taking in adolescence. Neuroimage 2013;71:275–83.

7. Grigg-Damberger MM. Ontogeny of sleep and its functions in infancy, childhood, and adolescence. In: Nevsimalova S, Bruni O, editors. Sleep disorders in chil-dren. Switzerland: Springer; 2017. p. 3–29.

8. Spruyt K. Neurocognitive effects of sleep disruption in children and adolescent. Child Adolesc Psychiatr Clin N Am 2021;30:27–45.

9. Liu X, Liu L, Owens JA, et al. Sleep patterns and sleep problems among school-children in the United States and China. Pediatrics 2005;115(1 suppl):241–9.

10. Meltzer LJ, Johnson C, Crosette J, et al. Prevalence of diagnosed sleep disorders in pediatric primary care practices. Pediatrics 2010;125(6):e1410–8.

11. Bruni O, Angriman M. Pediatric insomnia. In: Nevsimalova S, Bruni O, editors. Sleep disorders in children. Switzerland: Springer International Publishing; 2017.

12. Beebe DW. Cognitive, behavioral, and functional consequences of inadequate sleep in children and adolescents. Pediatr Clin North Am 2011;58(3):649–65.

13. Chervin RD, Dillon JE, Bassetti C, et al. Symptoms of sleep disorders, inattention, and hyperactivity in children. Sleep 1997;20:1185.

14. Ferber R. Solve your child's sleep problems. New York: Simon & Schuster; 2006.

15. Sheldon SAH, Ferber R, Kryger MH, et al. Principles and practice of pediatric sleep medicine. 2nd edition. New York: Elsevier Inc; 2014.

16. Honaker SM, Meltzer LJ. Sleep in pediatric primary care: a review of the literature. Sleep Med Rev 2016;25:31–9.

17. Lewandowski AS, Ward TM, Palermo TM. Sleep problems in children and adoles-cents with common medical conditions. Pediatr Clin North Am 2011;58(3):699–713.

18. Majde JA, Krueger JM. Links between the innate immune system and sleep. J Allergy Clin Immunol 2005;116(6):1188–98.

19. Fuligni AJ, Arruda EH, Krull JL, et al. Adolescent sleep duration, variability, and peak levels of achievement and mental health. Child Dev 2018;89(2):e18–28.

20. Gruber R, Carrey N, Weiss SK, et al. Position statement on pediatric sleep for psychiatrists. J Can Acad Child Adolesc Psychiatry 2014;23(3):174–95.

21. Meltzer LJ, et al. Clinical assessment of sleep. In: Meltzer LJ, Crabtree VM, edi-tors. Pediatric sleep problems: a clinician's guide to behavioral interventions. Washington, DC: American Psychological Association; 2015. p. 49-60.

22. Sheldon SH. Sleep history and differential diagnosis. In Sheldon SAH, Ferber R, Kryger MH, et al, editors. Principles and practice of pediatric sleep medicine. 2nd edition. New York: Elsevier Inc; 2014.

23. Harbard E, Allen NB, Trinder J, et al. What's keeping teenager up? Prebedtime behaviors and actigraphy-assessed sleep over school and vacation. J Adolesc Health 2016;58:426.

24. Perrault AA, Bayer L, Peuvrier M, et al. Reducing the use of screen electronic de-vices in the evening is associated with improved sleep and daytime vigilance in adolescents. Sleep 2019;42:zsz125.

25. Owens JA, Dalzell V. Use of the 'BEARS' sleep screening tool in a pediatric resident' continuity clinic: a pilot study. Sleep Med 2005;6:63.
26. Hamilton-Stubbs PE, Walters AS. Sleep disorders in children: simple sleep-related movement disorders. In: Nevsimalova S, Bruni O, editors. Sleep disorders in children. Switzerland: Springer; 2017. p. 227–51.
27. Cogen JD, Loghmanee DA. Sleep-related movement disorders. In In Sheldon SAH, Ferber R, Kryger MH, et al, editors. Principles and practice of pediatric sleep medicine. 2nd edition. New York: Elsevier Inc; 2014.
28. Prosperpio P, Nobili L. Parasomnias in children. In: Nevsimalova S, Bruni O, editors. Sleep disorders in children. Switzerland: Springer; 2017. p. 305–35.
29. Tan HL, Gozal D, Kheirandish-Gozal L. Obstructive sleep apnea in children: a short primer. In: Nevsimalova S, Bruni O, editors. Sleep disorders in children. Switzerland: Springer; 2017. p. 185–226.
30. Guilleminault C, Eldridge FL, Simmons FB, et al. Sleep apnea in eight children. Pediatrics 1997;58:23–30.
31. AAP (American Academy of Sleep Pediatrics) endorses new recommendations on sleep times. 2016. Available at: aappublications.org. https://www.aappublications.org/news/2016/06/13/Sleep061316. Accessed October 19, 2020.
32. Dewald JF, Meijer AM, Oort FJ, et al. The influence of sleep quality, sleep duration and sleepiness on school performance in children and adolescents: a meta-analytic review. Sleep Med Rev 2010;14(3):179–89.
33. Pasch KE, Iaska MN, Lytle LA, et al. Adolescent sleep, risk behaviors, and depressive symptoms: are they linked? Am J Health Behav 2010;34:237–48.
34. Roberts E, Roberts C, Duong HT. Sleepless in adolescence: prospective data on sleep deprivation, health and functioning. J Adolesc 2009;32:1045–57.
35. Gregory AM, Sadeh A. Sleep, emotional and behavioral difficulties in children and adolescents. Sleep Med Rev 2012;16(2):129–36.
36. Silva GE, Goodwin JL, Parthasarathy S, et al. Longitudinal association between short sleep, body weight, and emotional and learning problems in Hispanic and caucasian children. Sleep 2011;34:1197–205.
37. O'Brien LM, Mindell JA. Sleep and risk-taking behavior in adolescents. Behav *Sleep Med* 2005;3:113–33.
38. Tyagi V, Junega M, Rahul J. Sleep problems and their correlates in children with autism spectrum disorder: an Indian study. J Autism Dev Disord 2018;49:1169–81.
39. Ivanenko A, Kushnir J, Alfano CA. Sleep in psychiatric disorders. In: Sheldon SH, Ferber R, Kryger MH, et al, editors. Elsevier principles and practices of pediatric sleep medicine. Second edition. London: Sunders; 2014. p. 369–77.
40. Chan J, Edman JC, Koltai PJ. Obstructive sleep apnea in children. Am Fam Physician 2004;69(5):1147–55.
41. Sheldon SH, Ferber R, Kryger MH, et al. Principles and practices of pediatric sleep medicine. Second edition. London: Elsevier Saunders; 2014.
42. Nevsimalova S, Bruni O, editors. Sleep disorders in children. Switzerland: Springer; 2017.
43. Carter KA, Hathaway NE, Lettieri CE. Common sleep disorders in children. Am Fam Physician 2014;89(5):368–77.
44. Meltzer LJ, Crabtree VM. Pediatric sleep problems: a clinician's guide to behavioral interventions. Washington, DC: American Psychological Association; 2015.
45. Lunsford-Avery JR, Bidopia T, Jackson L, et al. Behavioral treatment of insomnia and sleep disturbances in school-aged children and adolescents. Child Adolesc Psychiatr Clin N Am 2021;30:101–16.

Sleep and Chronic Pain

Sleep Deficiency and Pediatric Chronic Pain

Shumenghui Zhai, MPH[a],*, Shameka Phillips, MSN, FNP-C[b], Teresa M. Ward, RN, PhD[c]

KEYWORDS

- Chronic pain • Sleep deficiency • JIA • Sickle cell • FGID • Evaluation • Treatment
- Children

KEY POINTS

- Children may be particularly vulnerable to the deleterious effects of sleep deficiency.
- Comorbid sleep deficiency in chronic pain may further exacerbate already existing symptoms of pain, anxiety, depressions, daytime function, and increase health care use.
- Routine sleep assessments and screening for sleep deficiency is necessary for children and adolescents with chronic pain conditions.
- Combining cognitive behavioral therapy for insomnia with human-centered design participatory approaches that partner with children, adolescents, and caregivers in the development of sleep interventions.
- This strategy can provide them with the knowledge, motivation, and skills for setting and achieving goals, adapting to setbacks, and problem solving, and shows great promise.

INTRODUCTION

An estimated 15% to 40% of children and adolescents suffer from pediatric chronic pain.[1] Chronic pain, defined as pain that occurs constantly or recurs frequently over a 3-month period, is costly to society, with estimates of $19.5 billion per year spent in the United States on health care costs.[1–3] Common pediatric chronic pain conditions include juvenile idiopathic arthritis (JIA), sickle cell disease (SCD), functional gastrointestinal disorders (FGIDs), and headaches (eg, migraines, tension headaches). Chronic pain is often comorbid with anxiety, depression, sleep deficiency, and fatigue, and interferes with daytime function, participation in school, sports and social activities, quality of life, and family functioning.[4–9] A history of childhood chronic pain places children at risk for a lifelong pattern of pain, disability, and high health care costs in adulthood.[10,11]

[a] University of Washington School of Nursing, Box 357266, Seattle, WA 98195, USA; [b] UAB Nutrition and Obesity Research Center (NORC), University of Alabama at Birmingham, School of Nursing, 1720 University Boulevard, Birmingham, AL 35294, USA; [c] Department of Child, Family, and Population Health Nursing, University of Washington School of Nursing, Box 357262, Seattle, WA 98195, USA
* Corresponding author.
E-mail address: sz69@uw.edu

Nurs Clin N Am 56 (2021) 311–323
https://doi.org/10.1016/j.cnur.2021.02.009   nursing.theclinics.com

Sleep deficiency, including inadequate quantity and poor quality of sleep, is highly comorbid in an estimated 50% of children and adolescents with chronic pain.[4,12] Studies have focused primarily on JIA, SCD, and migraines. Bedtime resistance, difficulty of falling asleep or maintaining sleep, short sleep duration, poor quality sleep (eg, feeling unrefreshed), and sleep-related anxiety are common self-report complaints. Short sleep duration, low sleep efficiency (eg, quality), bedtime variability, increased wake after sleep onset, and obstructive sleep apnea (OSA) as measured by actigraphy and polysomnography are also common.[13,14] Several studies have shown that sleep deficiency contributes to increased sensitivity to pain, impaired neurobehavioral performance, cardiovascular morbidity, poorer health-related quality of life, and increased health care use.[4,11–13,15,16]

INTERRELATIONSHIPS BETWEEN SLEEP AND PAIN

Complex bidirectional relationships exist between sleep, pain, physiology, mood, sociocontextual factors, and functional outcomes in pediatric chronic pain populations (**Fig. 1**). A biopsychosocial model suggests that pain occurs as a result of varying contributions from, and interactions between, biological, psychological, and social factors.[4] Sleep intersects with biology (eg, temperament), psychology (eg, mood, distress), and environment (eg, home, school, community). Early studies propose a bidirectional relationship between pain and sleep, such that sleep deficiency and pain reciprocally escalate over time.[17] Recent evidence suggests that sleep deficiency increases subsequent next-day pain in both experimental and self-report designs in multiple samples across childhood and adulthood.[4–6,13,14,18–21] Longitudinal studies have shown that poor quality and/or inadequate amounts of sleep is associated with new-onset pain, worsening pain and disability, depression, and poorer quality of life.[19] Further, several studies have also shown that insomnia may precede the onset of depression and chronic pain conditions.[22,23] A recent conceptualization of sleep deficiency by Harvey and colleagues[24] includes a transdiagnostic process that refers to the multiple causal factors or mechanisms that are common across medical and psychiatric conditions.[25]

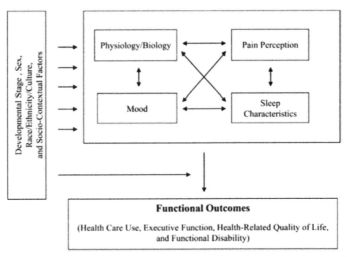

Fig. 1. Biopsychosocial model. (*From* Valrie CR, Bromberg MH, Palermo T, Schanberg LE. A Systematic Review of Sleep in Pediatric Pain Populations. J Dev Behav Pediatr JDBP. 2013;34(2):120-128. https://doi.org/10.1097/DBP.0b013e31827b5848.)

Less is known about the complex relations among sleep deficiency, pain, and sociocultural factors in relation to health disparities that adversely affects marginalized and disadvantaged pediatric populations.[26] For example, pediatric chronic pain populations who experience discrimination, are disadvantaged socioeconomically, lack access to health care, have gender identity differences (eg, lesbian, gay, bisexual, transgender, queer), and how these accumulative stressors intersect with biopsychosocial constructs and across individual, interpersonal, community, and societal levels is understudied.[27–31]

PEDIATRIC CHRONIC PAIN CONDITIONS
Headaches

An estimated 26% to 69% of children suffer from headaches (eg, migraines, tension, cluster).[1,4,32] Several studies show short sleep duration, poor sleep quality, insomnia, and sleep bruxism (eg, teeth grinding) in children and adolescents with headaches.[32–34] Prolonged headache duration and greater pain intensity and frequency have been shown to predict sleep anxiety, bedtime resistance, and sleep bruxism.[35–38] A recent retrospective chart review of pediatric children with chronic headache (n = 527 between 7 and 17 years of age) examined sleep disturbances and found that difficulties with sleep onset, frequent night awakenings, shorter sleep duration, and poor sleep hygiene were more common in children diagnosed with tension-type and daily persistent type headaches than those with migraines. Poorer sleep quality was associated inversely with functional disability, anxiety, and depression among children with tension-type headaches.[39]

Functional Gastrointestinal Disorders

FGIDs are among the most common abdominal problem, affecting 10% to 15% of children and adults.[40–42] FGIDs are characterized by persistent and intermittent abdominal pain without an identifiable organic cause. The severity of symptoms (eg, pain, vomiting) in children range from mild to severe and can be disabling.[43] The most common FGID is irritable bowel syndrome and functional abdominal pain.[44] FGIDs account for 50% of visits to pediatric gastroenterologists.[44] Sleep deficiency in children and adolescents with FGIDs is understudied,[9,45,46] despite studies in adult FGIDs that indicate sleep disruptions increase pain and symptom severity. Much of what is known about sleep deficiency in children rely on self-report, and difficulties with sleep onset and maintenance, poor quality, and daytime sleepiness are common.[9,11,45–48] Jansen and colleagues[48] examined sleep in 67 children with FGIDs, and found that 61% of 7- to 12-year-old children with FGIDs had sleep deficiency per parent report and poor sleep quality associated with pain-related interference. Two recent studies that measured sleep with actigraphy in school-age children reported a short sleep duration with an average total sleep time between 7.0 and 7.9 hours and poor sleep efficiency of between 82.3% and 84.0% in comparison with a community sample.[45]

Juvenile Idiopathic Arthritis

JIA is the most common pediatric rheumatologic condition characterized by joint pain, inflammation, and stiffness that interferes with physical mobility, well-being, and sleep.[49,50] Sleep deficiency is highly comorbid in children with JIA,[17,51–53] affecting an estimated 20% to 30% of children.[16,51,54] Difficulty falling asleep and returning to sleep, sleep anxiety, restless sleep, OSA, and daytime sleepiness are common parent- and child-reported sleep complaints. Short sleep duration and poor sleep quality owing to increased wake after sleep onset, restless sleep, and OSA have been shown by actigraphy and polysomnography.[5,14,15,23,55,56] Several studies have shown that increased pain is associated with sleep deficiency by both self-report and objective measures.[14,16,51–54,57]

Sickle Cell Disease

SCD is an inherited red blood cell disorder characterized by a lack of oxygen that results in abnormally shaped red blood cell and pain owing to blood vessel occlusion, ischemia, or infarction.[58–60] Pain and sleep disturbances including frequent night awakenings, difficulty falling asleep, daytime sleepiness, and sleep disorders (eg, OSA, periodic limb movement) have been reported in children with SCD.[4,55,58–61] The prevalence of OSA in SCD ranges from 5% to 79% based on findings from parent report and polysomnography.[4,55,58,61] OSA contributes to nocturnal hypoxemia and inflammation that has been linked to vaso-occlusive crises, pain, and acute chest syndrome.[56,58,61–63] In a large multicenter prospective study of 243 children with SCD, 41% had OSA, and habitual snoring (snoring >3 times a week) and lower oxygen saturation were the strongest predictors of OSA in children with SCD.[61]

COMMON SLEEP DISTURBANCES

Behavioral insomnia of childhood (BIC) includes bedtime resistance and difficulty of falling asleep or maintaining sleep that results in poor sleep quality and/or inadequate amounts of sleep.[64–67] An estimated 10% to 40% of children in the United States experience BIC at some point in childhood,[68] BIC includes 3 subtypes: (1) sleep-onset association type, (2) limit-setting type, and (3) BIC combined type.[69] Without proper treatment, BIC can persist into middle childhood and adolescence.

The sleep-onset association type of BIC type is characterized by the infant or toddler's lack of ability to self-soothing and dependency on specific parent intervention to fall asleep and to return to sleep after night awakenings.[70–73] For example, infants or toddlers who require parental presence (eg, falling asleep with feeding, being rocked or held to fall asleep, watching TV to fall asleep) to fall asleep and to return to sleep after a night awake.[65,68]

The limit-setting type of BIC includes bedtime refusal and/or bedtime stalling (eg, curtain calls)[65,66,74] and is common in children.[68,70] For example, children who ask for another glass of water, watch one more TV show, and/or use the computer before or at bedtime often experience prolonged (eg, delayed) sleep onset that can result in inadequate amounts of sleep. Likewise, children who have parents who fall asleep with them on some nights but refuse on other nights creates confusion for the child. Irregular and/or the lack of a consistent sleep routine and/or bedtime are often the culprits of limit-setting type of BIC.[70]

The combined type of BIC is the most common sleep problem for children and includes bedtime resistance in conjunction with frequent and problematic night waking.[64,66,71] For example, a child may refuse to go to bed (eg, temper tantrum) and/or has multiple curtain calls at bedtime, and then comes to the parents' bedroom in the middle of the night. In this condition, if parents react to the children's behavior by sleeping with them or allowing them to sleep in the parents' room, their behaviors will be reinforced.[66,74] Children with combined BIC struggle with both bedtime refusal and parental presence for sleep onset and sleep maintenance.

SLEEP DISORDERS

OSA is a sleep disorder characterized by complete or partial upper airway obstruction during sleep that disrupts gas exchange and ventilation.[72] The prevalence of OSA ranges from 1% to 5% in children and is increasing with a concomitant increase in childhood obesity.[72,73,75] OSA is associated with neurobehavioral deficits, cardiovascular morbidities (hypertension, obesity), impaired growth (failure to thrive), and poorer quality of life.[75] The peak age of OSA is between 2 and 6 years of age owing to the size of the tonsils and adenoids that can contribute to a decrease in the upper airway.[72,76] The risk factors for OSA include anatomic features (eg, enlarged adenoids and/or tonsils), obesity owing to excess tissue surrounding the upper airway that leads to a narrow airway, genetic disorders (eg, Down's syndrome, craniofacial underdevelopment, and cerebral palsy) that predispose children for increased upper airway collapsibility.[76,77] Additional risk factors for OSA include household smoking, asthma, and allergic rhinitis.[78,79] Prior studies report OSA in children with JIA, SCD, and FGID, and the underlying mechanisms may involve a combination of upper airway inflammation, craniofacial development, altered neurologic reflexes, and/or underlying inflammation.[33] Symptoms associated with OSA include snoring, observed pauses in breathing during sleep, restless sleep, enuresis, and unusual sleeping positions (eg, sleeping in an upright position and propped pillows). Children often present with noisy breathing, bedwetting, restless sleep (eg, tossing and turning), daytime sleepiness, and hyperactive, or inattentive daytime behavior. An overnight polysomnography is the gold standard to confirm the diagnosis of OSA.

Periodic limb movement disorder (PLMD) is a nocturnal movement disorder often associated with nocturnal sleep complaints and daytime sleepiness. Periodic limb movements usually involve the legs and are characterized as brief jerks of the limbs during sleep. Typically, PLMD is described as rhythmic extensions of the big toe and dorsiflexion of the ankle with occasional flexion of the knee and hip.[80] The diagnosis of PLMD is determined by polysomnography and a periodic limb movements index of greater than 5 per hour of sleep is considered abnormal.[81] PLMD has been reported in children with failure to thrive,[82,83] migraines,[33] juvenile fibromyalgia,[84] SCD,[55] and JIA.[85] Individual differences exist in the clinical presentation of children with PLMD. Symptoms may include sleepiness, insomnia, observed leg kicking during sleep, leg aches or pain in the morning, difficulty maintaining sleep and disrupted sleep, and daytime fatigue and tiredness.[82]

Insomnia is common in pediatric chronic pain conditions that affecting an estimated 27% to 54% of children and adolescents with chronic pain conditions report insomnia.[86–90] Insomnia subtypes include difficulty falling asleep, difficult maintaining sleep, and early morning awakening.[70] Insomnia is comorbid with anxiety, depression, and chronic pain conditions[86–90] and contribute to the onset of these symptoms.[22,23]

SLEEP ASSESSMENT

Routine sleep assessments are overlooked and not routinely assessed in children and adolescents with chronic pain conditions.[91] Conducting a thorough sleep assessment is time consuming and often challenging for clinicians who often have 15 minutes for a clinic visit. The BEARS[92] is a short practical sleep assessment tool that evaluates 5 domains of sleep (*Bedtime* issues, *Excessive* sleepiness, *Awakenings* during the night, *Regularity* and duration of sleep, and *Sleep*-disordered breathing) and includes questions specific to children 2 to 18 years old (**Table 1**). *Bedtime* issues refers to difficulties falling asleep and/or problems at bedtime and going to bed. Common bedtime problems include bedtime resistance, stalling, parental presence needed at bedtime, and/or media use at bedtime or in the bedroom. *Excessive* sleepiness refers to daytime sleepiness during school or while driving, being overly tired or sleepy during the day, and difficulty waking up in the morning. *Awakenings* during the night refers to

Table 1
BEARS sleep screening tool

	Toddler/Preschool (2–5 y)	School-Age (6–12 y)	Adolescent (13–18 y)
Bedtime problems	Does your child have any problems going to bed? Falling asleep?	Does your child have any problems at bedtime? (P) Do you have any problems going to bed? (C)	Do you have any problems falling asleep at bedtime? (C)
Excessive daytime sleepiness	Does your child seem overtired or sleepy a lot during the day? Does she still take naps?	Does your child have difficulty waking in the morning, seem sleepy during the day or take haps? (P) Do you feel tired a lot? (C)	Do you feel sleep a lot during the day? In school? While driving? (C)
Awakenings during the night	Does your child wake up a lot at night?	Does your child seem to wake up a lot at night? Any sleepwalking or nightmares? (P) Do you wake up a lot at night? Have trouble getting back to sleep? (C)	Do you wake up a lot at night? Have trouble getting back to sleep? (C)
Regularity and duration of sleep	Does your child have a regular bedtime and wake time? What are they?	What time does your child go to bed and get up on school days? Weekends? Do you think he/she is getting enough sleep? (P)	What time do you usually go to bed on school nights? Weekends? How much sleep do you usually get? (C)
Snoring	Does your child snore a lot or have difficulty breathing at night?	Does your child have loud or nightly snoring or any breathing difficulties at night? (P)	Does your teenager snore loudly or nightly? (P)

Abbreviations: (C), Child-directed question; (P), Parent-directed question.
Source: "A Clinical Guide to Pediatric Sleep: Diagnosis and Management of Sleep Problems" by Jodi A. Mindell and Judith A. Owens; Lippincott Williams & Wilkins.

number and frequency of nighttime awakenings and struggling to fall back asleep. *Regularity and duration of sleep* refers to a consistent sleep routine, bedtime and waketime, sleep duration, and the timing of sleep on the weekdays and weekends. *Sleep disordered breathing* refers to loud, noisy breathing while asleep, snoring, or difficulty breathing during sleep.

A thorough sleep history should include sleep–wake patterns on the weekday and weekends (eg, bedtime and wake time, regularity, satisfaction, timing), sleep environment (eg, varying sleep environments [different caregiver households], crowded living conditions), bedtime arrangement (eg, shared bed or bedroom), setup of the bedroom (eg, TV in the bedroom, media use, light, noise), daytime behavior (eg, hyperactive, inattentive, difficulty in concentrating, restlessness, daytime sleepiness), underlying comorbid symptoms (eg, pain, fatigue, anxiety, depression), child/family stress (eg, adverse childhood experiences, lack of resources [access to health care, socioeconomics, discrimination]), a family history of sleep disorders (eg, OSA, insomnia), and anatomic child/adolescent features (eg, tonsils and adenoids, retrognathia, high narrow palate, midfacial hypoplasia).[29,31,93,94] Children who struggle with falling asleep, restless sleep, sleep anxiety, or OSA may have daytime symptoms of hyperactivity, restlessness, inattentiveness, or fall asleep during school may be misdiagnosed with attention deficit hyperactivity disorder when the underlying problem is an inadequate amount of sleep and/or poor quality sleep.

TREATMENT OF SLEEP DEFICIENCY

Children and adolescents who screen positive for BIC and/or sleep disorders should be referred to a pediatric sleep specialist for further evaluation. For example, children who screen positive OSA may undergo lateral radiographs and/or upper airway MRI to assess the size of the tonsils and adenoids, and an overnight sleep study (eg, polysomnography), which is the gold standard to diagnose the severity of OSA. Mild OSA can be treated with topical nasal steroids, whereas moderate to severe OSA requires surgical intervention. A tonsillectomy and/or adenoidectomy is often the first line of treatment for moderate to severe OSA. Children who are refractive to surgical intervention often require noninvasive ventilation (eg, continuous positive airway pressure or bilevel positive airway pressure).

Cognitive behavioral therapy for insomnia (CBT-I) has been used to treat behavioral sleep problems in children and adolescents with chronic pain conditions.[87,95–98] CBT-I includes evidence-based practices that incorporate a multiple strategies such as sleep education, sleep skills training (eg, consistent sleep schedule, bedtime routine), lifestyle changes (eg, activities before bed), relaxation techniques, positive coping skills, communication, and parental strategies, such as reinforcement and modeling of positive coping skills, reward systems for activity participation, and communication with children that targets cognitive, behavioral, and social factors that may perpetuate insomnia, such as poor sleep hygiene practices (eg, too much time in bed), sleep anxiety (eg, rumination at bedtime), and negative attitudes about sleep (eg, concern about daytime deficits).[24,25,95] A recent pilot randomized controlled trial by Palermo and colleagues[87] tested the effectiveness of CBT-I in adolescents with chronic pain, insomnia, and comorbid physical or psychological difficulties, and found that CBT-I was associated with improved sleep hygiene, insomnia symptoms, and sleep quality both immediately after the intervention and at 3 months after the intervention. Symptoms of anxiety, depression, and health-related quality of life also improved. Currently, several investigators are using human-centered design approaches (HCA) to improve sleep and comorbid symptoms of pain, anxiety, and depression in pediatric chronic pain conditions.[95–99] HCA is a framework that integrates theory, research, practice, and end users into the design and development of products, and guides the creation of products or solutions to problems by engaging stakeholders throughout the entire design process. Involving stakeholders—children, adolescents, and caregivers—in the design and development ensures that a product solves pragmatic problems and addresses real-world user priorities and needs.[100] Integrating technology into CBT-I interventions decrease barriers for children, adolescents, families, and caregivers, such as long waiting lines, transportation to and from the clinic, missed work and school, lack of access to a pediatric sleep clinic, and financial concerns. HCA can be a powerful method in the development of web or mobile health based interventions to support the health of children, adolescents, and caregivers by providing tools to track and manage sleep.

SUMMARY

Given the prevalence of sleep deficiency in children and adolescents with chronic pain, routine assessments of sleep habits and screening for sleep deficiency is a critical component for the clinical care management of these children. Chronic pain is often comorbid with depression, anxiety, and sleep difficulties, and referrals to pediatric sleep clinics are often necessary owing to the need for CBT by trained pediatric sleep providers. Sleep deficiency is a modifiable behavior and partnering with both parents and children to provide them with the knowledge, motivation, and skills for setting and achieving goals, adapting to setbacks, and problem solving is essential. Although CBT-I has been shown to be an effective intervention to improve sleep in adults with chronic pain, and less in known about children and adolescents. Recent studies by Valrie, Palermo, and their colleagues have integrated HCA to improve sleep in children and adolescents with chronic pain show great promise.[87,97]

CLINICS CARE POINTS

- Sleep deficiency contributes to increased sensitivity to pain, mood disturbances, school absenteeism, lower health-related quality of life, and increased health care use.
- A thorough sleep assessment and sleep history should be conducted routinely in children and adolescents living with chronic pain.
- Referrals to pediatric sleep clinics are an excellent resource for health care providers who are unsure in how to manage and treat sleep deficiency in pediatric chronic pain.

DISCLOSURE

The authors have nothing commercial or financial conflicts of interest and any funding sources to disclose.

REFERENCES

1. King S, Chambers CT, Huguet A, et al. The epidemiology of chronic pain in children and adolescents revisited: a systematic review. Pain 2011;152(12): 2729–38.
2. Groenewald CB, Essner BS, Wright D, et al. The Economic costs of chronic pain among a cohort of treatment-seeking adolescents in the United States. J Pain 2014;15(9):925–33.
3. Maxion-Bergemann S, Thielecke F, Abel F, et al. Costs of irritable bowel syndrome in the UK and US. Pharmacoeconomics 2006;24(1):21–37.
4. Valrie CR, Bromberg MH, Palermo T, et al. A systematic review of sleep in pediatric pain populations. J Dev Behav Pediatr 2013;34(2):120–8.
5. Ward TM, Chen ML, Landis CA, et al. Congruence between polysomnography obstructive sleep apnea and the pediatric sleep questionnaire: fatigue and health-related quality of life in juvenile idiopathic arthritis. Qual Life Res 2017; 26(3):779–88.
6. Tsai S-Y, Labyak SE, Richardson LP, et al. Actigraphic sleep and daytime naps in adolescent girls with chronic musculoskeletal pain. J Pediatr Psychol 2008; 33(3):307–11.
7. Murphy LK, Palermo TM, Tham SW, et al. Comorbid sleep disturbance in adolescents with functional abdominal pain. Behav Sleep Med 2020;1–10. https://doi.org/10.1080/15402002.2020.1781634.

8. Nozoe KT, Polesel DN, Boin AC, et al. The role of sleep in Juvenile idiopathic arthritis patients and their caregivers. Pediatr Rheumatol 2014;12(1):20.
9. Schurman JV, Friesen CA, Dai H, et al. Sleep problems and functional disability in children with functional gastrointestinal disorders: an examination of the potential mediating effects of physical and emotional symptoms. BMC Gastroenterol 2012;12:142.
10. Walker LS, Dengler-Crish CM, Rippel S, et al. Functional abdominal pain in childhood and adolescence increases risk for chronic pain in adulthood. Pain 2010;150(3):568–72.
11. Varni JW, Bendo CB, Nurko S, et al. Health-related quality of life in pediatric patients with functional and organic gastrointestinal diseases. J Pediatr 2015; 166(1):85–90.
12. Badawy SM, Law EF, Palermo TM. The Interrelationship between sleep and chronic pain in adolescents. Curr Opin Physiol 2019;11:25–8.
13. Ward TM, Beebe DW, Chen ML, et al. Sleep disturbances and neurobehavioral performance in juvenile idiopathic arthritis. J Rheumatol 2017;44(3):361–7.
14. Yuwen W, Chen ML, Cain KC, et al. Daily sleep patterns, sleep quality, and sleep hygiene among parent–child dyads of young children newly diagnosed with juvenile idiopathic arthritis and typically developing children. J Pediatr Psychol 2016;41(6):651–60.
15. Beebe DW. Cognitive, behavioral, and functional consequences of inadequate sleep in children and adolescents. Pediatr Clin North Am 2011;58(3):649–65.
16. Butbul Aviel Y, Stremler R, Benseler SM, et al. Sleep and fatigue and the relationship to pain, disease activity and quality of life in juvenile idiopathic arthritis and juvenile dermatomyositis. Rheumatol Oxf Engl 2011;50(11):2051–60.
17. Lewin DS, Dahl RE. Importance of sleep in the management of pediatric pain. J Dev Behav Pediatr 1999;20(4):244–52.
18. Fisher K, Laikin AM, Sharp KMH, et al. Temporal relationship between daily pain and actigraphy sleep patterns in pediatric sickle cell disease. J Behav Med 2018;41(3):416–22.
19. Palermo TM, Law E, Churchill SS, et al. Longitudinal course and impact of insomnia symptoms in adolescents with and without chronic pain. J Pain 2012;13(11):1099–106.
20. Lewandowski AS, Palermo TM, De la Motte S, et al. Temporal daily associations between pain and sleep in adolescents with chronic pain versus healthy adolescents. Pain 2010;151(1):220–5.
21. Bromberg MH, Gil KM, Schanberg LE. Daily sleep quality and mood as predictors of pain in children with juvenile polyarticular arthritis. Health Psychol 2012; 31(2):202–9.
22. Baglioni C, Battagliese G, Feige B, et al. Insomnia as a predictor of depression: a meta-analytic evaluation of longitudinal epidemiological studies. J Affect Disord 2011;135(1):10–9.
23. Finan PH, Goodin BR, Smith MT. The association of sleep and pain: an update and a path forward. J Pain 2013;14(12):1539–52.
24. Harvey AG, Hein K, Dong L, et al. A transdiagnostic sleep and circadian treatment to improve severe mental illness outcomes in a community setting: study protocol for a randomized controlled trial. Trials 2016;17.
25. Treating sleep problems: a transdiagnostic approach. Guilford Press. Available at: https://www.guilford.com/books/Treating-Sleep-Problems/Harvey-Buysse/9781462531950. Accessed October 11, 2020.

26. National minority health and health disparities research framework. Available at: https://www.nimhd.nih.gov/about/overview/research-framework/.   Accessed October 5, 2020.

27. Hash JB, Oxford ML, Fleming CB, et al. Sleep problems, daily napping behavior, and social-emotional functioning among young children from families referred to child protective services. Behav Sleep Med 2020;18(4):447–59.

28. Hash JB, Oxford ML, Fleming CB, et al. Impact of a home visiting program on sleep problems among young children experiencing adversity. Child Abuse Negl 2019;89:143–54.

29. Sadler LS, Banasiak N, Canapari C, et al. Perspectives on sleep from multiethnic community parents, pediatric providers, and childcare providers. J Dev Behav Pediatr 2020;41(7):540–9.

30. Ordway MR, Sadler LS, Jeon S, et al. Sleep health in young children living with socioeconomic adversity. Res Nurs Health 2020;43(4):329–40.

31. Ward TM, Rankin S, Lee KA. Caring for children with sleep problems. J Pediatr Nurs 2007;22(4):283–96.

32. Dosi C, Figura M, Ferri R, et al. Sleep and headache. Semin Pediatr Neurol 2015;22(2):105–12.

33. Armoni Domany K, Nahman-Averbuch H, King CD, et al. Clinical presentation, diagnosis and polysomnographic findings in children with migraine referred to sleep clinics. Sleep Med 2019;63:57–63.

34. Esposito M, Parisi P, Miano S, et al. Migraine and periodic limb movement disorders in sleep in children: a preliminary case–control study. J Headache Pain 2013;14(1):57.

35. Palermo TM, Kiska R. Subjective sleep disturbances in adolescents with chronic pain: relationship to daily functioning and quality of life. J Pain 2005;6(3):201–7.

36. Carotenuto M, Guidetti V, Ruju F, et al. Headache disorders as risk factors for sleep disturbances in school aged children. J Headache Pain 2005;6(4):268–70.

37. Talebian A, Soltani B, Haji Rezaei M. Causes and associated factors of headaches among 5 to 15-year-old children referred to a neurology clinic in Kashan, Iran. Iran J Child Neurol 2015;9(1):71–5.

38. Heng K, Wirrell E. Sleep disturbance in children with migraine. J Child Neurol 2006;21(9):761–6.

39. Rabner J, Kaczynski KJ, Simons LE, et al. Pediatric headache and sleep disturbance: a comparison of diagnostic groups. Headache 2018;58(2):217–28.

40. Saps M, Seshadri R, Sztainberg M, et al. A prospective school-based study of abdominal pain and other common somatic complaints in children. J Pediatr 2009;154(3):322–6.

41. Everhart JE, Ruhl CE. Burden of digestive diseases in the United States part II: lower gastrointestinal diseases. Gastroenterology 2009;136(3):741–54.

42. Everhart JE, Ruhl CE. Burden of digestive diseases in the United States part I: overall and upper gastrointestinal diseases. Gastroenterology 2009;136(2):376–86.

43. Drossman DA, Morris CB, Schneck S, et al. International survey of patients with IBS: symptom features and their severity, health status, treatments, and risk taking to achieve clinical benefit. J Clin Gastroenterol 2009;43(6):541–50.

44. Hyams JS, Di Lorenzo C, Saps M, et al. Childhood functional gastrointestinal disorders: child/adolescent. Gastroenterology 2016;150(6):1456–68.e2.

45. Monzon AD, Cushing CC, Friesen CA, et al. The association between affect and sleep in adolescents with and without FGIDs. J Pediatr Psychol 2020;45(1): 110–9.

46. Gustafsson M-L, Laaksonen C, Salanterä S, et al. Associations between daytime sleepiness, psychological symptoms, headache, and abdominal pain in school-children. J Sch Nurs 2019;35(4):279–86.

47. Varni JW, Lane MM, Burwinkle TM, et al. Health-related quality of life in pediatric patients with irritable bowel syndrome: a comparative analysis. J Dev Behav Pediatr 2006;27(6):451–8.

48. Jansen J, Ward T, Levy RL, et al. Sa1622 Sleep disturbances in school-age children with functional gastrointestinal pain disorders and relation to demographic and clinical characteristics. Gastroenterology 2020;158(6):S-357.

49. Ravelli A, Martini A. Juvenile idiopathic arthritis. Lancet 2007;369(9563):767–78.

50. Eisenstein EM, Berkun Y. Diagnosis and classification of juvenile idiopathic arthritis. J Autoimmun 2014;48-49:31–3.

51. Ward TM, Yuwen W, Voss J, et al. Sleep fragmentation and biomarkers in juvenile idiopathic arthritis. Biol Res Nurs 2016;18(3):299–306.

52. Ward TM, Sonney J, Ringold S, et al. Sleep disturbances and behavior problems in children with and without arthritis. J Pediatr Nurs 2014;29(4):321–8.

53. Lopes MC, Guilleminault C, Rosa A, et al. Delta sleep instability in children with chronic arthritis. Braz J Med Biol Res 2008;41(10):938–43.

54. Shyen S, Amine B, Rostom S, et al. Sleep and its relationship to pain, dysfunction, and disease activity in juvenile idiopathic arthritis. Clin Rheumatol 2014; 33(10):1425–31.

55. Rogers VE, Marcus CL, Jawad AF, et al. Periodic limb movements and disrupted sleep in children with sickle cell disease. Sleep 2011;34(7):899–908.

56. Salles C, Ramos R, Daltro C, et al. Prevalência da apneia obstrutiva do sono em crianças e adolescentes portadores da anemia falciforme. J Bras Pneumol 2009;35. https://doi.org/10.1590/S1806-37132009001100004.

57. Bromberg MH, Connelly M, Anthony KK, et al. Self-reported pain and disease symptoms persist in juvenile idiopathic arthritis despite treatment advances: an electronic diary study. Arthritis Rheumatol 2014;66(2):462–9.

58. Katz T, Schatz J, Roberts CW. Comorbid obstructive sleep apnea and increased risk for sickle cell disease morbidity. Sleep Breath Schlaf Atm 2018;22(3): 797–804.

59. Valrie CR, Trout KL, Bond KE, et al. Sleep problem risk for adolescents with sickle cell disease: sociodemographic, physical, and disease-related correlates. J Pediatr Hematol Oncol 2018;40(2):116–21.

60. Ramos-Machado V, Ladeia AM, Dos Santos Teixeira R, et al. Sleep disorders and endothelial dysfunction in children with sickle cell anemia. Sleep Med 2019;53:9–15.

61. Rosen CL, Debaun MR, Strunk RC, et al. Obstructive sleep apnea and sickle cell anemia. Pediatrics 2014;134(2):273–81.

62. Hankins JS, Verevkina NI, Smeltzer MP, et al. Assessment of sleep-related disorders in children with sickle cell disease. Hemoglobin 2014;38(4):244–51.

63. Dlamini N, Saunders DE, Bynevelt M, et al. Nocturnal oxyhemoglobin desaturation and arteriopathy in a pediatric sickle cell disease cohort. Neurology 2017; 89(24):2406–12.

64. Brown S, Johnston B, Amaria K, et al. A randomized controlled trial of amitriptyline versus gabapentin for complex regional pain syndrome type I and neuropathic pain in children. Scand J Pain 2016;13(1):156–63.

65. Owens JA, Moore M. Insomnia in infants and young children. Pediatr Ann 2017; 46(9):e321–6.
66. Moore M. Behavioral sleep problems in children and adolescents. J Clin Psychol Med Settings 2012;19(1):77–83.
67. Moore M. Bedtime problems and night wakings: treatment of behavioral insomnia of childhood. J Clin Psychol 2010;66(11):1195–204.
68. Nunes ML, Bruni O. Insomnia in childhood and adolescence: clinical aspects, diagnosis, and therapeutic approach. J Pediatr (Rio J) 2015;91(6 Suppl 1): S26–35.
69. Sateia MJ. International classification of sleep disorders-third edition. Chest 2014;146(5):1387–94.
70. Owens JA, Mindell JA. Pediatric insomnia. Pediatr Clin North Am 2011;58(3): 555–69.
71. Meltzer LJ. Clinical management of behavioral insomnia of childhood: treatment of bedtime problems and night wakings in young children. Behav Sleep Med 2010;8(3):172–89.
72. Marcus CL, Brooks LJ, Draper KA, et al. Diagnosis and management of childhood obstructive sleep apnea syndrome. Pediatrics 2012;130(3):576–84.
73. Arens R, Muzumdar H. Childhood obesity and obstructive sleep apnea syndrome. J Appl Physiol (1985) 2010;108(2):436–44.
74. Carter KA, Hathaway NE, Lettieri CF. Common sleep disorders in children. Am Fam Physician 2014;89(5):368–77.
75. Dehlink E, Tan H-L. Update on paediatric obstructive sleep apnoea. J Thorac Dis 2016;8(2):224–35.
76. Chang SJ, Chae KY. Obstructive sleep apnea syndrome in children: epidemiology, pathophysiology, diagnosis and sequelae. Korean J Pediatr 2010; 53(10):863–71.
77. Bitners AC, Arens R. Evaluation and management of children with obstructive sleep apnea syndrome. Lung 2020;198(2):257–70.
78. Weinstock TG, Rosen CL, Marcus CL, et al. Predictors of obstructive sleep apnea severity in adenotonsillectomy candidates. Sleep 2014;37(2):261–9.
79. Marcus CL, Moore RH, Rosen CL, et al. A randomized trial of adenotonsillectomy for childhood sleep apnea. N Engl J Med 2013;368(25):2366–76.
80. Durmer JS, Quraishi GH. Restless legs syndrome, periodic leg movements, and periodic limb movement disorder in children. Pediatr Clin North Am 2011;58(3): 591–620.
81. Aurora RN, Lamm CI, Zak RS, et al. Practice parameters for the non-respiratory indications for polysomnography and multiple sleep latency testing for children. Sleep 2012;35(11):1467–73.
82. Picchietti MA, Picchietti DL. Restless legs syndrome and periodic limb movement disorder in children and adolescents. Semin Pediatr Neurol 2008; 15(2):91–9.
83. Cielo CM, DelRosso LM, Tapia IE, et al. Periodic limb movements and restless legs syndrome in children with a history of prematurity. Sleep Med 2017;30: 77–81.
84. Tayag-Kier CE, Keenan GF, Scalzi LV, et al. Sleep and periodic limb movement in sleep in juvenile fibromyalgia. Pediatrics 2000;106(5):E70.
85. Ward TM, Archbold K, Lentz M, et al. Sleep disturbance, daytime sleepiness, and neurocognitive performance in children with juvenile idiopathic arthritis. Sleep 2010;33(2):252–9.

86. Clarke G, McGlinchey EL, Hein K, et al. Cognitive-behavioral treatment of insomnia and depression in adolescents: a pilot randomized trial. Behav Res Ther 2015;69:111–8.
87. Palermo TM, Beals-Erickson S, Bromberg M, et al. A single arm pilot trial of brief cognitive behavioral therapy for insomnia in adolescents with physical and psychiatric comorbidities. J Clin Sleep Med 2017;13(3):401–10.
88. Law EF, Wan Tham S, Aaron RV, et al. Hybrid cognitive-behavioral therapy intervention for adolescents with co-occurring migraine and insomnia: a single-arm pilot trial. Headache 2018;58(7):1060–73.
89. Palermo TM, Wilson AC, Lewandowski AS, et al. Behavioral and psychosocial factors associated with insomnia in adolescents with chronic pain. Pain 2011; 152(1):89–94.
90. Kanstrup M, Holmström L, Ringström R, et al. Insomnia in paediatric chronic pain and its impact on depression and functional disability. Eur J Pain 2014; 18(8):1094–102.
91. Ward TM. Chapter 5. Conducting a sleep assessment. In: Redeker N, McEnany G, Phillips, editros. Sleep disorders and sleep promotion in nursing practice. 1st edition. New York: Springer; 2011. p. 53-70.
92. Owens JA, Dalzell V. Use of the "BEARS" sleep screening tool in a pediatric residents' continuity clinic: a pilot study. Sleep Med 2005;6(1):63–9.
93. Ordway MR, Wang G, Jeon S, et al. Role of sleep duration in the association between socioecological protective factors and health risk behaviors in adolescents. J Dev Behav Pediatr 2020;41(2):117–27.
94. Lee KA, Ward TM. Critical components of a sleep assessment for clinical practice settings. Issues Ment Health Nurs 2005;26(7):739–50.
95. Ward TM, Skubic M, Rantz M, et al. Human-centered approaches that integrate sensor technology across the lifespan: opportunities and challenges. Nurs Outlook 2020. https://doi.org/10.1016/j.outlook.2020.05.004.
96. Yuwen W, Backonja U, Bromberg M, et al. Participatory design of a web-based intervention for parents to improve sleep in young children with arthritis. In AMIA. 2019.
97. Valrie CR, Kilpatrick RL, Alston K, et al. Investigating the sleep-pain relationship in youth with sickle cell utilizing mHealth technology. J Pediatr Psychol 2019; 44(3):323–32.
98. Birnie KA, Campbell F, Nguyen C, et al. iCanCope PostOp: user-centered design of a smartphone-based app for self-management of postoperative pain in children and adolescents. JMIR Form Res 2019;3(2):e12028.
99. Sonney J, Duffy M, Hoogerheyde LX, et al. Applying human-centered design to the development of an asthma essentials kit for school-aged children and their parents. J Pediatr Health Care 2019;33(2):169–77.
100. Eikey EV, Reddy MC, Kuziemsky CE. Examining the role of collaboration in studies of health information technologies in biomedical informatics: a systematic review of 25 years of research. J Biomed Inform 2015;57:263–77.

Moving?

Make sure your subscription moves with you!

To notify us of your new address, find your **Clinics Account Number** (located on your mailing label above your name), and contact customer service at:

Email: journalscustomerservice-usa@elsevier.com

800-654-2452 (subscribers in the U.S. & Canada)
314-447-8871 (subscribers outside of the U.S. & Canada)

Fax number: 314-447-8029

**Elsevier Health Sciences Division
Subscription Customer Service
3251 Riverport Lane
Maryland Heights, MO 63043**

*To ensure uninterrupted delivery of your subscription, please notify us at least 4 weeks in advance of move.